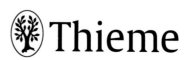 Thieme

Treatment of Oral Diseases

A Concise Textbook

George Laskaris, M.D., D.D.S., Ph.D.

Head of Oral Medicine, Department of
Dermatology, A. Sygros Hospital
Associate Professor of Oral Medicine
Medical School, University of Athens
Athens, Greece
Visiting Professor
University of London, UK

Thieme
Stuttgart · New York

Library of Congress Cataloging-in-Publication Data

Laskaris, George.
Treatment of oral diseases : a concise textbook / Georg Laskaris ; with contributions by P. Angelakis ... [et al.]. p. ; cm.
Companion v. to: Color atlas of oral diseases / George Laskaris. 3rd ed., rev. and expanded. c2003.
Includes bibliographical references.
ISBN 3-13-130111-2 (GTV : alk. paper) –
ISBN 1-58890-176-9 (TNY : alk. paper)
1. Mouth–Diseases.
[DNLM: 1. Mouth Diseases–diagnosis. 2. Mouth Diseases–drug therapy. 3. Mouth Diseases–therapy. WU 166 L344t 2005] I. Angelakis, Philip. II. Laskaris, George. Enchromos atlas stomatologias. English. III. Title.

RC815.L3733 2005
616.3'106–dc22

2004018493

© 2005 Georg Thieme Verlag,
Rüdigerstrasse 14, 70469 Stuttgart, Germany
http://www.thieme.de

Thieme New York, 333 Seventh Avenue,
New York, NY 10001 USA
http://www.thieme.com

Cover design: Martina Berge, Erbach
Typesetting by Satzpunkt Ewert GmbH, Bayreuth
Printed in Germany by Druckhaus Götz, Ludwigsburg
ISBN 3-13-130111-2 (GTV)
ISBN 1-58890-176-9 (TNY)   1 2 3 4 5

Dedication

This book is dedicated to the brightest star,
my son **Christos G. Laskaris**,
whose memory leads my mind and life

Preface

Oral medicine is an important discipline and the diagnostic and therapeutic challenges faced by the stomatologist range from trivial, isolated, innocuous oral lesions to the oral manifestations of life-threatening systemic diseases. It requires a thorough understanding of and a firm knowledge base in dentistry, oral pathology, otorhinolaryngology, dermatology, and internal medicine.

The diagnostic part of the practice of oral medicine is addressed in many excellent texts including the *Color Atlas of Oral Diseases* by the author of this volume.

This book aims to provide a concise, practical, and reliable guide to the management of oral diseases. The field of therapeutics of oral diseases is progressing rapidly and every effort has been made to include evidence-based multimodality therapeutic regimens—drugs, surgery, and other therapeutic means—where appropriate. However, I ask the reader to keep in mind that this book is not meant to be a substitute for a thorough knowledge base or the comprehensive literature on each and every therapeutic component used in clinical practice. Nor is it aiming to present details of surgical techniques.

The emphasis is on formulating and implementing a sound therapeutic plan, following an initial clinical evaluation, a comprehensive differential diagnosis, and an accurate final diagnosis. Three universal principles of therapeutics are highlighted. The first principle of management of oral disease is comprehensive and addresses the patient as a whole, not just a particular lesion. The time devoted to establishing a healthy and trusting relationship with the patient and his patient's family, alleviating anxiety, fear and other concerns, explaining the pros and cons of various therapeutic strategies in simple terms, is time well spent for both the patient and the phy-

sician. Secondly, in complex problems, cooperation and consultation among the various subspecialties involved in the care of a patient, with clearly defined roles and goals for all involved, are mandatory. Lastly, since the time of Hippocrates, therapeutic excess leading to harm is to be avoided—in modern terms, the choice of a particular therapeutic approach should be based on the available scientific evidence.

The book is divided into three parts: Part I presents the definition and a brief summary of each disease—etiology, main clinical features, diagnosis and differential diagnosis, and a detailed multimodality treatment plan. For practical purposes, disease entities appear in alphabetical order in the contents. Part II provides information regarding the main categories of drugs and the commonly used individual drugs within these categories, which have proved useful in the treatment of a particular disease. Part III provides a synopsis of the basic principles and oral applications of lasers, which are making significant inroads in the field of oral therapeutics.

It is my hope that stomatologists, oral surgeons, dentists, dermatologists, otorhinolaryngologists, pediatricians, and internists alike will find the information in the book useful for the treatment of oral diseases.

Sincere thanks are due to the contributors of this volume for sharing their experience and knowledge of the treatment of specific oral diseases. I would also like to express my gratitude and thanks to Dr Stathis S Papavasiliou, Associate Professor of Internal Medicine, for his helpful comments and corrections. Finally, my deepest gratitude goes to my family for their constant support and love.

Athens, September 2004   *George Laskaris*

List of Contributors

Philip Angelakis, M.D., D.M.R.T., F.R.C.R. (UK)
Head Department of Radiation Oncology
Hygeia Hospital
Athens, Greece
(Radiotherapy of Squamous Cell Carcinoma)

Nikos Choulis, Ph.D. (London)
Professor of Pharmacy
University of Athens
Athens, Greece
(Drugs)

Eleni Gagari, D.M.D., D.M.Sc.
Associate Professor of Oral and Maxillofacial
Pathology
School of Dental Medicine
Tufts University
Boston, MA, USA
(Chemical Burn, Thermal Burn, Drug-Related Mucosal Pigmentation, Epulis Fissuratum, Metal Deposition, Nicotinic Stomatitis, Smoker's Melanosis, Smokeless Tobacco Keratosis)

John Iatrou, D.D.S., M.D., Ph.D.
Associate Professor of Oral and Maxillofacial
Surgery
Dental School
University of Athens
Athens, Greece
(Surgical Treatment of Squamous Cell Carcinoma)

Chrysostomos Melissinos, M.D., Ph.D.
Pneumonologist
Hygeia Hospital
Athens, Greece
(Treatment of Tuberculosis)

Gerassimos Pangalis, M.D., Ph.D.
Professor of Hematology
Medical School
University of Athens
Athens, Greece
(Treatment of Leukemias and non-Hodgkin-Lymphomas)

George E. Romanos, D.D.S., D.M.D., Dr. med. dent., Ph.D.
Professor of Implant Dentistry
College of Dentistry
New York University
New York, N.Y., U.S.A.
(Laser Therapy)

George Stathopoulos, M.D., Ph.D.
Medical Oncologist
Director of Oncology Clinic
E. Dunant Hospital
Athens, Greece
(Chemotherapy of Squamous Cell Carcinoma)

George Vaiopoulus, M.D., Ph.D.
Professor of Internal Medicine
Medical School
University of Athens
Athens, Greece
(Treatment of Amyloidosis)

Contents

Abbreviations

BP	bullous pemphigold
CT	computed tomography
Dsg	desmoglein
FAPA	(periodic) fever, aphthous ulcers, pharyngitis, adenitis
GM-CSF	Granulocyte-macrophage colony-stimulating factor
HCV	hepatitis C virus
HIV	human immune deficiency virus
HPV	human papillomavirus
HSV	herpes simplex virus
i. m.	intramuscular
i.v.	intravenous
MIC	minimum inhibitory concentration
MIU	million international units
MU	million units
NSAIDs	nonsteroidal anti-inflammatory drugs
PCR	polymerase chain reaction
RAU	recurrent aphthous ulcers
rhG-CSF	recombinant human granulocyte colony-stimulating factor
s. c.	subcutaneous
TNF	tumor necrosis factor
U	units
VSV	varicella zoster virus

Important Points

- Before treatment an accurate diagnosis of each disease entity must be made.
- Treatment without prior diagnosis is, as a rule, unsuccessful and may be dangerous for the patient.
- Medicines must be prescribed only when they are necessary and when the benefits have been considered in relation to the risks involved.
- For treatment to be successful the choice of the correct drug and the patient's compliance with the physician's instructions are necessary.
- Clinicians must thoroughly understand, for every drug, the mechanism of action, clinical indications, interactions, side effects, formulations, and the dosage.
- Almost all drugs have several side effects on multiple organ systems.
- Physicians should choose the treatment with the optimal outcome and reasonable cost.
- New drugs must be used with caution.

- Stomatologists and dentists should avoid undertaking the treatment of the systemic diseases presenting with oral manifestations. The treatment of these diseases must be provided by the respective specialists.
- Topical treatment of oral manifestations of systemic diseases must always be undertaken in collaboration with the patient's physician.
- Several serious oral diseases require hospital care.
- There should be a good rapport or understanding between the physician and the patient—it is important for most therapeutic measures to be effective.

"Ωφελέειν εἰ μή βλάττειν"
("To benefit, or do not harm")
(Hippocrates, 460–377 BC)

This must always be in the mind of the physician before making decisions about diagnosis and treatment.

Part I
Diseases

Actinic Cheilitis

▦ Definition

Actinic cheilitis is a relatively common precancerous disorder typically confined to the vermilion zone of the lower lip.

▦ Etiology

Fair-skinned individuals with high occupational or recreational sun exposure are more commonly affected.

▦ Main Clinical Features

- Chronic mild edema and erythema followed by dryness and fine scaling
- The epithelium becomes progressively thin and atrophic with hyperkeratotic whitish papules or small plaques intermingled with red areas
- Later the lip becomes very dry and scaly with erosions
- Risk of development of leukoplakia and squamous cell carcinoma is increased

▦ Diagnosis

The clinical diagnosis should be confirmed by a biopsy and histopathologic examination.

▦ Differential Diagnosis

- Leukoplakia
- Discoid lupus erythematosus
- Lichen planus
- Scleroderma
- Contact cheilitis
- Herpes simplex
- Cheilitis due to radiation
- Squamous cell carcinoma

▦ Treatment

Basic Guidelines

- Sun-protective measures should always be recommended.
- Patients should use lip lubricants containing sunscreens.
- Before treatment, a biopsy is necessary to determine histologic changes.
- Periodic follow-up is necessary because of the increased risk of malignant transformation.

Suggested Therapies

- Nonsurgical procedures are recommended for patients without epithelial dysplasia or invasive squamous cell carcinoma
  - Topical 5-fluorouracil cream (0.5–5%) may be applied once or twice daily for 2–3 weeks. However, because of local irritation and relatively poor results this treatment is not included in the first-line therapies.
  - Recently, the topical immunomodulator, imiquimod cream 5% (Aldara) has been used successfully for the treatment of actinic cheilitis. The suggested regimen is to apply two or three times weekly for 4–6 weeks. Local adverse reactions such as erythema, edema, and erosions may occur. Systemic adverse effects, e.g., fever, headache, fatigue, diarrhea, and myalgia may occur in 1–2% of patients.
  - Carbon dioxide (CO_2) laser ablation has also been used for the treatment of actinic cheilitis with excellent results.
- Surgical treatment is recommended for patients with epithelial dysplasia, carcinoma in situ, or invasive squamous cell carcinoma. Vermilionectomy is the treatment of choice in such cases.

Alternative Therapies

Alternative therapies include photodynamic therapy, i.e., application of 5-aminolevulinic acid followed by exposure to a light source, and cryosurgery. Both methods are indicated for patients without premalignant or malignant foci histologically. Radiation therapy has also been used with success.

References

Dufresne RG, Curlin MU. Actinic cheilitis: A treatment review. *Dermatol Surg* 1997;3:15–21.

Ishida CE, Ramos-e-Silva M. Cryosurgery in oral lesions. *Int J Dermatol* 1998;37:283–285.

Kaugars GE, Pillion T, Svirsky JA, et al. Actinic cheilitis. A review of 152 cases. *Oral Surg Oral Med Oral Pathol Oral Radiol Endod* 1999;88:181–186.

Picascia DD, Robinson JK. Actinic cheilitis: A review of the etiology, differential diagnosis and treatment. *J Am Acad Dermatol* 1987;17:255–264.

Smith KJ, Germain M, Yeager J, Skclton II. Topical 5% imiquimod for the therapy of actinic cheilitis. *J Am Acad Dermatol* 2002;47:497–501.

Vega-Memije ME, Mosqueda-Taylor A, Irigoyen-Camacho ME, et al. Actinic prurigo cheilitis: Clinicopathologic analysis and therapeutic results in 116 cases. *Oral Surg Oral Med Oral Pathol Oral Radiol Endod* 2002;94:83–91.

Zelickson BD, Roenigk RK. Actinic cheilitis. Treatment with the carbon dioxide laser. *Cancer* 1990;5:1307–1311.

Actinomycosis

Definition

Actinomycosis is a chronic granulomatous infectious disease.

Etiology

Actinomycosis is caused by the anaerobic Gram-positive bacterium *Actinomyces israelii* and rarely by other species.

Classification

There are three main clinical types: a) cervicofacial, b) thoracic, and c) abdominal.

Main Clinical Features

Cervicofacial actinomycosis is the most common type (about 50–60% of cases) of the disease and oral lesions form a part of it. The infection typically follows dental infection, tooth extraction, or trauma to the oral mucosa.

Oral Manifestations

- Painless, slow-growing, hard swelling—the classic features of cervicofacial actinomycosis
- Multiple abscesses draining to the surface by sinus tracts. Yellow purulent material representing colonies of *Actinomyces* (sulfur granules) may discharge from the sinuses
- Scar formation
- New abscesses and sinuses may develop
- Jaw and salivary gland involvement is common
- Trismus is common
- Periapical inflammatory lesions may also occur
- Tongue, buccal mucosa, lips, gingiva, and tonsils are the most common oral sites involved

Diagnosis

The clinical diagnosis should be confirmed by biopsy and histopathologic examination, direct microbiologic examination and culture, and indirect immunofluorescence.

Differential Diagnosis

- Periodontal abscess
- Dental abscess
- Tuberculosis
- Systemic mycoses
- Other infections
- Benign and malignant tumors

Treatment

Basic Guidelines

- The response to treatment is slow.
- Treatment should be continued for weeks or months after clinical cure to avoid recurrences.
- The best therapeutic regimen includes a combination of drugs and surgery.

Suggested Therapies

- Intramuscular penicillin G, 10–20 MU/day for 4–6 weeks, is the drug of choice for early cervicofacial actinomycosis. This regimen is usually followed by oral penicillin V 500 mg four times daily for 1–3 months. Localized, limited disease usually responds well to a combination of surgical removal of the infected tissues and a 2–4-week course of penicillin.
- Tetracycline 500 mg three to four times daily for 2–4 months may be used as an alternative drug for patients allergic to penicillin.
- Intramuscular or intravenous ampicillin 50 mg/kg per day for 4–6 weeks, followed by oral amoxicillin 500 mg/day for 6–12 additional months should be given to prevent recurrences.
- Surgical procedures such as drainage and resection should be also carried out along with the drug therapy for better results.

Alternative Therapy

Sulfamethoxazole 2–4 g/day for 4–6 weeks or more is an alternative regimen.

References

Hirshberg A, Tsesis I, Metzger Z, Kaplan I. Periapical actinomycosis: A clinicopathologic study. *Oral Surg Oral Med Oral Pathol Oral Radiol Endod* 2003;95:614–620.

Laskaris G. Oral manifestations of infectious diseases. *Dent Clin North Am* 1996;40:395–423.

Rahnama M, Tomaszewski T. Cervicofacial actinomycosis: An issue still present. *Ann Univ Mariae Curie Sklodowska* 2001;56:447–449.

Rush JR, Sulte HR, Cohen DM, Makkawy H. Course of infection and case outcome in individuals diagnosed with microbial colonies morphologically consistent with *Actinomyces* species. *J Endod* 2002;28:613–618.

Adenocarcinomas of the Salivary Glands

▣ Definition

Salivary gland adenocarcinomas constitute a relatively rare group of oral malignancies originating from the epithelium of the major or minor salivary glands.

▣ Etiology

The etiology of adenocarcinomas of the salivary glands is unknown.

▣ Classification

- Mucoepidermoid carcinoma
- Adenoid cystic carcinoma
- Malignant pleomorphic adenoma
- Acinic cell adenocarcinoma
- Clear cell adenocarcinoma
- Polymorphous low-grade adenocarcinoma
- Adenocarcinoma not otherwise specified
- Epithelial-myoepithelial carcinoma
- Other types

▣ Main Clinical Features

The box gives the clinical features of minor salivary gland malignant neoplasms only.

- Slow-growing, usually painless, rubbery swelling
- Tumor may be slightly mobile and may ulcerate later
- Size progressively increases and pain may develop during the late stages
- Soft palate, buccal mucosa, and upper lip are the most commonly affected sites
- Clinical features are not characteristic and diagnostic

▣ Diagnosis

The clinical diagnosis should be confirmed by biopsy and histopathologic examination.

▣ Differential Diagnosis

- Different types of malignant salivary gland tumor
- Pleomorphic adenoma
- Monomorphic adenoma
- Mucocele
- Necrotizing sialadenometaplasia
- Non-Hodgkin lymphoma
- Malignant granuloma
- Squamous cell carcinoma
- Sarcomas

▣ Treatment

Basic Guidelines

- Before treatment a full clinical examination and laboratory investigations should be done.
- The treatment depends on the grade and stage of each tumor.
- A follow-up program is necessary as recurrences and metastasis are relatively common.
- Details of the surgical procedures are beyond the scope of this book.

Suggested Therapies

- Radical surgical excision is the treatment of choice in all types of malignant salivary gland neoplasms.
- Postoperative radiation therapy may also be used as adjuvant therapy in advanced and aggressive neoplasms.

References

Bensdoum RJ, Allavena C, Chauvel P, et al. 2003 update of standards, options and recommendations for radiotherapy for patients with salivary gland malignant tumors. *Cancer Radiother* 2003;7:280–295.

Brandwein MS, Ivanov K, Wallace DI, et al. Mucoepidermoid carcinoma: a clinicopathologic study of 80 patients with special reference to histological grading. *Am J Surg Pathol* 2001;25:835–845.

Caccamese JF, Ord RA. Paediatric mucoepidermoid carcinoma of the palate. *Int J Oral Maxillofac Surg* 2002;31: 136–139.

Castle JT, Thompson LD, Frommelt RA, et al. Polymorphous low grade adenocarcinoma: a clinicopathologic study of 164 cases. *Cancer* 1999;6:207–219.

Darling MR, Schneider JW, Phillips VM. Polymorphous low-grade adenocarcinoma and adenoid cystic carcinoma: a review and comparison of immunohistochemical markers. *Oral Oncol* 2002;38:641–645.

Laskaris G. *Color Atlas of Oral Diseases*, 3rd edition. Thieme Verlag: Stuttgart, 2003.

Neville BW, Damm DD, Allen CM, Bouquot JE. *Oral and Maxillofacial Pathology*, 2nd edition. WB Saunders Co.: Philadelphia, 2002.

Agranulocytosis

▨ Definition

Agranulocytosis is a hematologic disorder characterized by a severe reduction or absence of granulocytes, in particular, the neutrophils ($<500/mm^3$).

▨ Etiology

Agranulocytosis may be caused by drug treatment and infections, although some cases are idiopathic.

▨ Main Clinical Features

Oral lesions mainly occur early in the disease and are common.

Oral Manifestations

- Necrotic ulcers covered by a gray-white pseudomembrane without a red halo
- Increased salivation and painful mastication are common symptoms
- Severe necrotizing gingivitis with destruction of periodontal tissues may occur

Systemic Manifestations

- Sudden chills, fever, malaise, and sore throat
- Within 12–24 hours, signs and symptoms of respiratory, and/or gastrointestinal, or other bacterial infections often develop
- Risk of infections is usually related to the degree of neutropenia

▨ Diagnosis

The clinical diagnosis should be confirmed by a complete blood count and bone marrow aspiration.

▨ Differential Diagnosis

- Neutropenia
- Cyclic neutropenia
- Aplastic anemia
- Acute leukemia
- Infectious mononucleosis
- Wegener granulomatosis
- Acute necrotizing ulcerative gingivitis and stomatitis

▨ Treatment

Basic Guidelines

- Potential causative drug must be discontinued.
- High level of oral hygiene must be maintained.
- Any dental and gingival treatment during the acute phase of the disease should be avoided.
- The systemic treatment must be provided by a specialist.

Suggested Therapies

Topical Treatment

The use of mouthwashes such as 0.1% chlorhexidine gluconate and oxygen peroxide may reduce the severity of the oral lesions.

Systemic Treatment

- Systemic administration of appropriate broad-spectrum antibiotics in doses and duration proportional to the severity of the bacterial infection.
- Granulocyte-macrophage colony-stimulating factor (GM-CSF) or recombinant human granulocyte colony-stimulating factor (rhG-CSF) is effective in shortening the recovery time in patients with agranulocytosis.

References

Friedman I, Klepfish A, Miller EB, et al. Agranulocytosis in Sjögren's syndrome: Two case reports and analysis of 11 additional reported cases. *Semin Arthritis Rheum* 2002;31:338–345.

Welte K, Dale D. Pathophysiology and treatment of severe chronic neutropenia. *Ann Hematol* 1996;72:158.

Amalgam Tattoo

Definition

Amalgam tattoo is a common pigmented lesion of the oral mucosa.

Etiology

The tattoo is caused by implantation of amalgam particles in the oral mucosa.

Main Clinical Features

- Gray, black, or bluish macular or papular lesion that is usually solitary, although patients may also present with multiple lesions
- The lesion may be visible radiographically as a radio-opacity, provided that the amalgam particles are large enough

Diagnosis

The diagnosis is usually based on clinical criteria.

Differential Diagnosis

- Other types of tattoos
- Pigmented nevi
- Malignant melanoma
- Racial pigmentation
- Hematoma
- Addison disease

Treatment

No treatment is necessary, unless aesthetics are a concern. In this case, tissue resurfacing surgery may be done.

References

Forsell M, Larsson B, Ljungqvist A, et al. Mercury content in amalgam tattoos of human oral mucosa and its relation to local tissue reactions. *Eur J Oral Sci* 1998;106:582–587.

Stewart CM, Watson RE. Experimental oral foreign body reactions. Commonly employed dental materials. *Oral Surg Oral Med Oral Pathol* 1990;69:713–719.

Amyloidosis

Definition

Amyloidosis is a rare metabolic disorder characterized by an abnormal extracellular deposition of amyloid, a fibrillar proteinaceous material, in tissues.

Etiology

The etiology of amyloidosis is not fully understood.

Classification

Four major types of amyloidosis are recognized: primary, secondary, familial, and senile. Primary and secondary amyloidosis may be either systemic or localized.

Main Clinical Features

The oral mucosa is usually involved (30–50%) in primary systemic amyloidosis, while oral lesions are rare in the secondary form.

Oral Lesions

- Petechiae, ecchymoses, papules, nodules, swellings
- Macroglossia, ulcers
- Salivary gland infiltration
- Xerostomia and rarely bullae
- The deep red hue is characteristic of all oral lesions

Skin Lesions

- Purpura, petechiae, papules, nodules, macules
- Ulcers, hemorrhage, bullae
- Alopecia
- Waxy discoloration of the skin
- Periorbital ecchymoses

Systemic Manifestations

- Fatigue, weakness, weight loss, edema, dyspnea, hoarseness, bleeding, pain
- Carpal tunnel syndrome
- Heart, renal, joints, skeletal muscles, gastrointestinal tract, nervous system and other organ involvement
- Multiple myeloma may be associated with 10–20% of cases of primary systemic amyloidosis

Diagnosis

The clinical diagnosis should be confirmed by a biopsy and histopathologic examination with special stains (Congo red, methyl violet, thioflavine T).

Differential Diagnosis

- Lipoid proteinosis
- Sarcoidosis
- Crohn disease
- Multiple neurofibromatosis
- Lupus vulgaris
- Pemphigus
- Bullous pemphigoid
- Macroglossia due to other causes

Treatment

Basic Guidelines

- There is no specific therapy.
- The treatment is usually aimed at alleviating the symptoms and does not lead to removal of the amyloid deposits.
- The treatment of oral lesions is also symptomatic and usually unsuccessful.
- Amyloidosis must be treated by a specialist.

Suggested Therapies

Topical Treatment

- High level of oral hygiene is necessary.
- Topical corticosteroids and immunomodulators (e. g., tacrolimus) are useful, particularly in cases with oral ulcerations.
- Antiseptic rinses may be used in cases of infection of oral lesions.

Systemic Treatment

Primary Amyloidosis

Primary amyloidosis (AL), in particular of the kidney, is treated with alkylating agents (e.g., melphalan) and corticosteroids. This treatment can reduce the proteinuria and improve renal function in a few patients. The administration of a new anthracycline (4'-iodo-4'-deoxydoxorubicin) can also induce rapid improvement in some patients. The effectiveness of anthracycline is attributed to the binding of the drug to the amyloid fibrils. Bleeding diathesis can be treated with high-dose melphalan chemotherapy and autologous bone marrow transplantation.

Secondary Amyloidosis

Secondary amyloidosis (AA) with renal or hepatic involvement due to familial Mediterranean fever is treated with colchicine 0.6 mg twice daily, which prevents or arrests further progression of the disease process. In patients with chronic hemodialysis-related amyloidosis, renal transplantation is considered. Renal transplantation is also an option in patients with secondary amyloidosis. Adequate control of inflammation early in the course of rheumatoid arthritis may prevent the development of secondary amyloidosis or slow the progression of organ failure if this complication has already developed. Cytotoxic drugs (e.g., chlorambucil) may reduce the frequency of AA.

Alternative Therapies

Dimethyl sulfoxide (DMSO), which may partially dissolve amyloid fibrils has been shown to be effective in some patients with AA, but the resultant body odor makes it unacceptable and thus currently it is only used topically in patients with extensive cutaneous amyloidosis. A new approach to the treatment of systemic amyloidosis and other diseases associated with local amyloid is with a new compound called carboxy-pyrrolidin-oxo-hexanoyl pyrrolidine-carboxylic acid (CPHPC). This is a competitive inhibitor of serum amyloid P component (SAP) binding to amyloid fibrils, resulting in the removal of SAP from amyloid deposits in the tissues.

References

Baxbaum J. The amyloidoses. In: Klippel JH, Dieppe PA (eds). *Rheumatology*, 2nd edition. Mosby: London, 1998: pp.8.27.1–18.27.10.

Cunnane G, Whitehead AS. Amyloid precursors and amyloidosis in rheumatoid arthritis. *Bailliere's Clin Rheumatol* 1999;13:615–628.

Haukins PN. Hereditary systemic amyloidosis with renal involvement. *J Nephrol* 2003;16:443–448.

Merlini G, Anesi E, Garini P, et al. Treatment of AL amyloidosis with 4'-iodo-4'-deoxydoxorubicin: An update. Blood 1999;93:1112–1113.

Pepys MB, Herbert J, Hutchinson WL, et al. Targeted pharmacological depletion of serum amyloid P component for treatment of human amyloidosis. *Nature* 2002;417: 254–259.

Skinner M, Sanchorawala V, Seldin DC, et al. High-dose melfalan and autologous stem-cell transplantation in patients with AL amyloidosis: An 8-year study. Ann Intern Med 2004;140:85–93.

Stoopler ET, Sollecito TP, Chen SY. Amyloid deposition in the oral cavity: A retrospective study and review of the literature. *Oral Surg Oral Med Oral Pathol Oral Radiol Endod* 2003;95:674–680.

Suhr OB, Svendsen IH, Andersson R, et al. Hereditary transthyretin amyloidosis from a Scandinavian perspective. *J Intern Med* 2003;254:225–235.

Angina Bullosa Hemorrhagica

■ Definition

Angina bullosa hemorrhagica is a rare, acute, benign, oral disorder characterized by blood-filled blisters.

■ Etiology

The etiology is unknown. However, mild mucosal trauma and long-term use of inhaled corticosteroids have been implicated in the pathogenesis.

■ Main Clinical Features

- Single or multiple hemorrhagic bullae that soon rupture leaving a superficial ulcer
- Ulcer usually heals spontaneously without scarring in 5–10 days
- Soft palate and rarely, the buccal mucosa and the tongue are the areas of predilection
- Older individuals are more frequently affected

■ Diagnosis

The diagnosis is based mainly on the medical history and the clinical features. Biopsy, histopathologic examination, and direct immunofluorescence may be used to rule out other bullous diseases.

■ Differential Diagnosis

- Cicatricial pemphigoid
- Bullous pemphigoid
- Linear IgA disease
- Epidermolysis bullosa acquisita
- Oral amyloidosis
- Blood dyscrasias

■ Treatment

Basic Guidelines

- Patients should avoid hard foods.
- If the patient is using inhaled corticosteroids the patient's internist or physician should be consulted before any treatment is prescribed.

Suggested Therapies

- Usually the lesions regress in a few days without any treatment.
- However, when multiple lesions appear, systemic oral corticosteroids, e.g., prednisone 10–20 mg/day for 1 week helps to heal the ulcerations sooner. This is important as multiple lesions may produce severe discomfort and pain.
- The use of mouthwashes with oxygen releasing agents (3 % hydrogen peroxide), is recommended for multiple lesions in connection with corticosteroids.

References

De las Heras ME, Moreno R, Nunez M, et al. Angina bullosa hemorrhagica. *J Dermatol* 1996;23:507–509.
Grinspan D, Abulafia J, Lanfranchi H. Angina bullosa hemorrhagica. *Int J Dermatol* 1999;38:525–528.
Guillot B. Skin reactions to inhaled corticosteroids. Clinical aspects, incidence, avoidance, and management. *Am J Clin Dermatol* 2000;1:107–111.
Stephenson P, Lamey PJ, Scully C, et al. Angina bullosa hemorrhagica: clinical and laboratory features in 30 patients. *Oral Surg Oral Med Oral Pathol* 1987;63:560–565.

Angiocentric T-cell Lymphoma

Definition

Angiocentric T-cell lymphoma, nasal natural killer (NK)/T-cell lymphoma, malignant granuloma, or midline lethal granuloma is a rare aggressive form of lymphoma characteristically involving the midline structures of the palate and nasal cavity.

Etiology

The etiology is unknown, although the Epstein–Barr virus is frequently associated with this form of lymphoma.

Main Clinical Features

- Prodromal signs and symptoms, e.g., epistaxis, pain, and nasal stuffiness
- Swelling, nonhealing ulceration, and necrosis of the palate, alveolar processes, retromolar pads and the nasal cavity are common, causing destruction and perforation of the palate, nasal septum and bones
- Secondary infections and hemorrhage usually complicate the course of the disease

Diagnosis

The clinical diagnosis should be confirmed by biopsy and histopathologic examination and immunohistochemical evaluation.

Differential Diagnosis

- Wegener granulomatosis
- Non-Hodgkin lymphoma
- Squamous cell carcinoma
- Necrotizing sialadenometaplasia
- Mucormycosis
- Other multiple mycoses
- Leprosy
- Syphilitic gumma

Treatment

Suggested Therapies

- High-dose radiation therapy is the treatment of choice, in particular, of localized early disease. The lesion usually responds well to this treatment and recurrences are rare.
- Chemotherapy alone or in combination with radiation must be used for aggressive and disseminated disease. The prognosis of this form is unfavorable.

References

Koch M, Blatterspiel GJ, Niedobitek G, Konstantinidis J. Angiocentric T/NK cell lymphoma: A special clinical-pathological entity of lethal midline granuloma. A case report. *Laryngorhinootologie* 2001;80:410–415.

Lee PY, Freeman NJ, Khorsand J, et al. Angiocentric T-cell lymphoma presenting as lethal midline granuloma. *Int J Dermatol* 1997;36:419–427.

Mosqueda-Taylor A, Meneses-Garcia A, Zarate-Osorno A, et al. Angiocentric lymphomas of the palate: Clinico-pathological consideration in 12 cases. *J Oral Pathol Med* 1997;26:93–97.

Torre V, Bucolo S, Galletti B, Cavallari V. Midfacial granuloma syndrome or an inflammatory non-specific disease? *J Oral Pathol Med* 2001;30:190–192.

Vidal E, Dean A, Alamillos F, et al. Lethal midline granuloma in a human immunodeficiency virus-infected patient. *Am J Med* 2001;111:244–245.

Angular Cheilitis

■ Definition

Angular cheilitis or perlèche is a common inflammatory disorder of the corners of the mouth.

■ Etiology

Angular cheilitis has a multifactorial etiology. Systemic diseases (anemia, diabetes mellitus, human immunodeficiency virus [HIV] infection), xerostomia, habitual licking of the corners of the mouth, reduced vertical dimension of the face, and local infection by *Candida albicans, Staphylococcus aureus* and streptococci are the most common causes.

■ Main Clinical Features

- Maceration, erythema, fissuring, erosions, and crusting at the commissures
- Saliva tends to pool at the corners of the mouth, keeping them moist and favoring *Candida* and bacterial infection
- Lesions are usually painful

■ Diagnosis

The diagnosis is based on the clinical features.

■ Treatment

Basic Guidelines

- Before any topical treatment the presence of a systemic disease should be ruled out. In cases with an underlying disease, control of the disease improves the angular cheilitis as well.
- If loss of vertical dimension is the cause it must be corrected by the dentist.

Suggested Therapies

- Application of a topical ointment with corticosteroids, antimycotics, and antibacterial agents, two to three times daily for 1–2 weeks improves the condition dramatically.
- Topical treatment with nystatin or imidazole ointment is helpful but not always curative.
- Systemic triazoles, e.g., itraconazole capsules 100 mg/day for 6 days or more, are necessary if oral candidiasis is diagnosed.

References

Appleton SS. Candidiasis: pathogenesis, clinical characteristics and treatment. *J Calif Dent Assoc* 2000;28:942–948.

Kuffer R, Husson C. Superficial and angular cheilitis. *Ann Dermatol Venereol* 2000;127:88–92.

Ohman SC, Dahlen G, Moller A, Ohman A. Angular cheilitis: A clinical and microbial study. *J Oral Pathol* 1986;15: 213–217.

Ohman SC, Jontell M, Dahlen G. Recurrence of angular cheilitis. *Scand J Dent Res* 1988;96:360–365.

Rose AJ. Aetiology of angular cheilosis. *BDJ* 1968;125:67.

Aphthous Ulcers

▣ Definition and Epidemiology

Recurrent aphthous ulcers (RAU) or recurrent aphthous stomatitis (RAS) are painful oral ulcerations that characteristically recur at intervals ranging from days to months or even years. They represent the most common lesion of the oral mucosa with an overall prevalence ranging from 15% to 30%. Females are more commonly affected than males. Although the lesions may appear at any age, they usually present during the second and third decades of life. Familial occurrence is common and about 30–40% of the patients with RAU have another affected family member.

▣ Etiology

RAU is one of the oldest oral diseases, to be known since the time of Hippocrates, yet its etiology still remains unclear. Many predisposing factors have been incriminated such as genetics, trauma, food hypersensitivities, stress, infections (*Streptococcus sanguis* and *S. mitis,* herpes simplex virus [HSV]-1, varicella zoster virus [VZV], cytomegalovirus), and systemic factors. Although predisposing factors may play a role in the development of RAU the disease is idiopathic and its etiology remains unknown. Accumulated data support the concept that the pathophysiology of RAU is immunologically mediated, and involves dysregulation of the cell-mediated immune response.

▣ Main Clinical Features

Based on clinical criteria, recurrent aphthae are classified into minor, major, and herpetiform ulcers (Table **1**).

Table 1.1 Clinical features of the three types of aphthous ulcer

Type	Diameter	Number	Duration	Scarring
Minor	3–6 mm	1–6	6–10 days	No
Major	1–2 cm	1–3	3–6 weeks	Yes, rarely
Herpetiform	1–3 mm	10–100	10–15 days	No

The main clinical features of the three forms are painful, recurrent oral ulcerations at intervals ranging from days to weeks or even months. The prodromal stage is variable and is usually characterized by discomfort and occasionally erythema of 1–3 days duration. This stage is soon followed by a painful oral ulcer.

The lesions are usually confined to movable nonkeratinized or poorly keratinized oral mucosa, e.g., buccal mucosa, labial mucosa, tongue, floor of the mouth, soft palate, and uvula.

Clinicians should bear in mind that RAU may be associated with several systemic disorders.

Systemic Disorders Associated with RAU

- Behçet disease
- Sweet syndrome
- Crohn disease
- Ulcerative colitis
- Celiac disease
- HIV infection
- Malabsorption syndromes
- Hematinic deficiencies
- Neutropenia
- FAPA syndrome

▣ Diagnosis

The diagnosis of all three forms of RAU is based exclusively on clinical criteria, as there is no specific test, unless there is an underlying systemic disease.

▣ Differential Diagnosis

- Traumatic ulcer
- Primary and secondary herpetic stomatitis
- Hand, foot, and mouth disease
- Herpangina
- Stomatitis medicamentosa
- Erythema multiforme
- Pemphigus
- Pemphigoid
- Syphilis (chancre and mucous patches)

- Behçet disease
- Crohn disease
- Ulcerative colitis
- Cyclic neutropenia

▒ Treatment

Basic Guidelines

- When managing RAU, it is important to rule out aphthous-like ulcers associated with systemic diseases. The great majority of patients with RAU are healthy individuals with no history or signs of systemic disease.
- Successful therapy of RAU requires correct diagnosis and control of the contributing etiologic factors.
- A wide spectrum of therapeutic regimens or agents has been recommended, but the management of RAU is unsatisfactory, as there is no cure and all attempts at treatment are palliative.
- The goal of treatment should be a) elimination of pain and discomfort, b) shortening of the course of the disease, and c) avoiding recurrences.

Suggested Therapies

- Control of the contributing etiologic factors
- Topical treatment
- Systemic treatment

Control of Possible Contributing Etiologic Factors

Patients should be encouraged to keep a food diary in an attempt to identify a potential precipitating link with the onset of aphthous ulcers. Patients should avoid minor trauma of the oral mucosa. Stress and female sex hormonal fluctuations should also be monitored and if possible controlled. A gluten-free diet may be useful in controlling lesions even in the absence of celiac disease.

Topical Treatment

Topical medications may reduce pain and shorten the course, but they do not prevent recurrence.

Topical anesthetics such as 2% viscous lidocaine, benzocaine, and benzydamine hydrochloride may reduce pain only for a short time. Recently, 5% amlexanox oral paste and 3% diclofenac in 2.5% hyaluronan have also been employed to reduce pain with partial success. Topical tetracyclines have also been used with partial success. A 250 mg capsule is dissolved in 30 ml of water, and 5 ml of this solution is used to rinse the lesion four to six times a day. This is repeated for 3–5 days. Many other anti-inflammatory and antimicrobial agents (chlorhexidine, listerine) have also been used with unsatisfactory results. The most effective topical agents are 0.1% triamcinolone acetonide in an oral adhesive base (Orabase), 0.5% fluocinonide gel (Lidex gel) or 0.05% clobetasol propionate gel (Temovate) applied to the ulcer three to six times a day for 4–6 days. Intralesional injection of triamcinolone acetonide retard or betamethasone dipropionate and sodium phosphate retard may be successful for major aphthous ulcers only.

Systemic Treatment

Systemic corticosteroids (prednisone and betamethasone in an average dose of 20–30 mg and 2–3 mg, respectively) for 4–8 days are very helpful for major ulcers or herpetiform ulcers. In cases of repeated episodes and when new ulcers occur before the previous ones have healed, systemic medications may prove useful in preventing new lesions. In our experience, 20 mg prednisone or 2 mg betamethasone for 10–15 days and then an injection of betamethasone dipropionate and sodium phosphate retard (Celestone Chronodose) every 2 weeks for a period of 2 months may significantly increase the periods between recurrences. Long-term systemic corticosteroids are contraindicated because of their side effects.

In severe cases with a high recurrence rate and in HIV-infected patients, thalidomide 100–300 mg/day for 2–3 months may result in complete remission of the ulcers for a long time. However, teratogenesis and polyneuropathy preclude the routine use of thalidomide.

Clinicians should be aware that safe prophylaxis for prevention of recurrences of RAU in the long term is not possible.

Alternative Therapies

In severe cases many other systemic medications have been used with ambiguous results. These include dapsone, levamisole hydrochloride, colchicine, azathioprine, interferon alpha, cyclosporine, pentoxifylline, and recently rebamipide, a gastroprotective drug.

References

Ball SC, Sepkowitz KA, Jacobs JL. Thalidomide for treatment of oral aphthous ulcers in patients with human immunodeficiency virus: Case report and review. *Am J Gastroenterol* 1997;92:169–170.

Brown RS, Bottomley WK. Combination immunosuppressant and topical steroid therapy for treatment of recurrent major aphthae. *Oral Surg Oral Med Oral Pathol* 1990,69:42–44.

Fontes V, Machet L, Huttenberger B, et al. Recurrent aphthous stomatitis: Treatment with colchicine. An open trial of 54 cases. *Ann Dermatol Venereol* 2002;129:1365–1369.

Haeyrinen-Immonen R, Sorsa T, Pettilae J, et al. Effect of tetracyclines on collagenase activity in patients with recurrent aphthous ulcers. *J Oral Pathol Med* 1994;23:269–272.

Laskaris G. *Color Atlas of Oral Diseases*, 3rd edition. Thieme: Stuttgart, 2003.

Laskaris G. Aphthous stomatitis. In: Katsambas A, Lotti TM (eds). *European Handbook of Dermatological Treatments*. Springer: Berlin, 2003.

MacPhail L. Topical and systemic therapy for recurrent aphthous stomatitis. *Semin Cutan Med Surg* 1997;16:301.

Matsuda T, Ohno S, Hirohata S, et al. Efficacy of rebamipide as adjunctive therapy in the treatment of recurrent oral aphthous ulcers in patients with Behçet's disease: A randomised, double-blind placebo-controlled study. *Drugs R D* 2003;4:19–28.

Paterson DL, Georghiou PR, Allworth AM, Kemp RJ. Thalidomide as treatment of refractory aphthous ulceration related to human immunodeficiency virus infection. *Clin Infect Dis* 1995;20:250–254.

Rees TD, Binnie WH. Recurrent aphthous stomatitis. *Dermatol Clin* 1996;14:243–256.

Scully C, Porter SR. Recurrent aphthous stomatitis: Current concepts of etiology, pathogenesis and management. *J Oral Pathol Med* 1989,18:21–27.

Vincent SD, Lilly GE. Clinical, historic, and therapeutic features of aphthous stomatitis. *Oral Surg Oral Med Oral Pathol* 1992;74:79–86.

Woo SB, Sonis ST. Recurrent aphthous ulcers: A review of diagnosis and treatment. *JADA* 1996;127:1202–1213.

Ariboflavinosis

▨ Definition

Ariboflavinosis or vitamin B_2 deficiency is an unusual disorder that usually occurs in combination with other vitamin deficiencies.

▨ Etiology

Deficiency of vitamin B_2 occurs due to dietary inadequacy, achlorhydria, malabsorption, alcoholic cirrhosis, hypothyroidism, and drugs.

▨ Main Clinical Features

Oral Manifestations

- Angular cheilitis
- Atrophy of the filiform papillae resulting in a smooth red tongue
- Dry and cracked lips

Other Manifestations

- Skin lesions include perioral seborrheic dermatitis, scaly papules, fissures, and, rarely, ulcers
- Conjunctivitis and photophobia
- Anemia, mental disorders, and slowing of higher functions; weakness may occur

▨ Diagnosis

The diagnosis is based mainly on the medical history and clinical features. Biochemical analysis of vitamin B_2 status and measurement of erythrocyte glutathione reductase helps confirm the diagnosis.

▨ Differential Diagnosis

- Pellagra
- Plummer–Vinson syndrome
- Other vitamin B complex deficiencies
- Zinc deficiency
- Angular cheilitis

▨ Treatment

Basic Guidelines

- Improve or treat any underlying illness.
- Eat foods rich in vitamin B_2 (meat, fish).

Suggested Therapies

- Treatment consists of riboflavin 5–15 mg/day taken orally until the clinical signs and symptoms are resolved. In severe cases 2–4 mg two times daily can be given parenterally.
- Topical antifungals such as nystatin or miconazole ointment may be used for the treatment of angular cheilitis.
- A high level of oral hygiene is necessary.

References

Barthelemy H, Chouvet B, Cambazard F. Skin and mucosal manifestations in vitamin deficiency. *J Am Acad Dermatol* 1986;15:1263.

Mataix J, Aranda P, Sanchez C, et al. Assessment of thiamin (vitamin B_2) status in an adult Mediterranean population. *Br J Nutr* 2003;90:661–666.

Miller SJ. Nutritional deficiency and the skin. *J Am Acad Dermatol* 1989;21:1–30.

Roe DA. Riboflavin deficiency: Mucocutaneous signs of acute and chronic deficiency. *Semin Dermatol* 1991;10: 293–7.

Aspergillosis

Definition

Aspergillosis is an opportunistic fungal infection with a broad spectrum of clinical manifestations.

Etiology

Aspergillus fumigatus and *A. flavus* are the main pathogenic *Aspergillus* species. Immunocompromised patients such as those with HIV infection, neutropenia, leukemia, and diabetes, those receiving immunosuppressant agents and organ transplantation, and patients with chronic respiratory diseases are more susceptible to *Aspergillus* infection.

Classification

There are several types of *Aspergillus* infection: a) allergic aspergillosis, b) aspergilloma (fungus balls), c) invasive aspergillosis (pulmonary involvement in 90–95% and extrapulmonary involvement in 20–25%), d) chronic necrotizing pulmonary aspergillosis, and e) superficial aspergillosis with skin, ear, and eye involvement.

Main Clinical Features

The oral mucosa is usually affected in invasive pulmonary aspergillosis. Rarely, the oral lesions are the initial manifestation of the disease.

Oral Manifestations

The oral lesions present as irregular ulcers with a typical yellowish-black surface due to necrosis of the tissues. The lesions are usually localized to the palate, tongue, and lips

Invasive Pulmonary Aspergillosis

Fever, cough, dyspnea, retrosternal and pleuritic pain, and tachycardia are the most common symptoms and signs. However, many patients with invasive pulmonary aspergillosis are asymptomatic

Diagnosis

Oral lesions should be biopsied and histopathologically examined. A computed tomography (CT) scan of the chest for suspected pulmonary infection is recommended. Bronchoscopy, biopsy, and respiratory cultures can also be useful.

Differential Diagnosis

- Histoplasmosis
- Mucormycosis
- Cryptococcosis
- Other systemic mycoses
- Agranulocytosis
- Squamous cell carcinoma
- Non-Hodgkin lymphoma
- Malignant granuloma
- Wegener granulomatosis

Treatment

Basic Guidelines

- The treatment of oral lesions of aspergillosis must be undertaken in collaboration with the specialist.
- Invasive pulmonary aspergillosis is one of the most difficult diseases to treat and mortality is high.
- Early diagnosis and early initiation of antifungal treatment are important for a successful outcome.
- Remission and control of the underlying disease are important for a favorable prognosis.
- Relapse may occur.
- The treatment of aspergillosis is always systemic.

Suggested Therapies

- Intravenous amphotericin B is the first-line drug for invasive aspergillosis. The drug must be given only by specialists in a hospital unit.
- Oral itraconazole is an important agent in the treatment of all types of aspergillosis. A dose of 200–400 mg/day is given for weeks to months depending on the type and the sever-

ity of the disease. In addition, itraconazole oral solution 5 mg/kg per day is effective.

- Corticosteroids are used only for allergic aspergillosis.

Future Therapies

Voriconazole and caspofungin seem to be effective in invasive aspergillosis. However, more clinical trials are needed.

References

Andriole VT. *Aspergillus* infections: Problems in diagnosis and treatment. *Infect Agent Dis* 1996;5:47.

Johnson LB, Kauffman CA. Voriconazole: A new triazole antifungal agent. *Clin Infect Dis* 2003;36:630–637.

Kontoyiannis DP, Bodey GP. Invasive aspergillosis in 2002: An update. *Eur J Clin Microbiol Infect Dis* 2002;21:161–172.

Koss T, Bagheri B, Zeama C, et al. Amphotericin B-resistant, *Aspergillus flavus* infection successfully treated with caspofungin, a novel antifungal agent. *J Am Acad Dermatol* 2002;46:945–947.

Letscher-Bru V, Herbecht R. Caspofungin: The first representation of a new antifungal class. *J Antimicrob Chemother* 2003;51:513–521.

Myoken Y, Sugata T, Kyo T, et al. Itraconazole prophylaxis for invasive gingival aspergillosis in neutropenic patients with acute leukemia. *J Periodontol* 2002;73:33–88.

Rubin AI, Bagheri B, Scher RK. Six novel antimycotics. *Am J Clin Dermatol* 2002;3:71–81.

Bacillary Angiomatosis

■ Definition

Bacillary angiomatosis is a recently described uncommon tumor-like bacterial infection.

■ Etiology

The causative organisms are *Bartonella henselae* and *quintana*. The disease usually affects patients in advanced stages of HIV infection (CD$_4$+ lymphocytes <50 cells/mm^3) and rarely other immunocompromised patients or patients with malignancies.

■ Main Clinical Features

Visceral, skin, and oral lesions may occur.

Oral Lesions

- Asymptomatic, dark red, slightly elevated nodule or tumor
- Soft on palpation
- Gingiva, palate, and tongue are most commonly affected

Skin Lesions

- Dark red and violaceous papules and nodules
- Usually painless
- Subcutaneous nodules which may erode the skin surface

Constitutional Symptoms

- Fever, malaise, night sweats
- Lymphadenopathy
- Abdominal pain
- Hepatosplenomegaly
- Anemia

■ Diagnosis

The diagnosis should be confirmed by biopsy and histologic examination.

■ Differential Diagnosis

- Kaposi sarcoma
- Pyogenic granuloma
- Pregnancy granuloma
- Peripheral giant cell granuloma
- Hemangioma
- Leiomyoma
- Brown giant cell tumor
- Other vascular tumors

■ Treatment

Basic Guidelines

- Oral bacillary angiomatosis should be regarded as an important marker for predicting the progression of HIV infection.
- Treatment is always systemic.
- Surgical excision of solitary lesions is usually not necessary.

Suggested Therapies

- Erythromycin 500 mg four times daily, or azithromycin 250 mg daily, or clarithromycin 500 mg twice daily is the drug of choice for bacillary angiomatosis. The treatment should continue for 6–8 months.
- Oral doxycycline 100 mg twice daily or oral ciprofloxacin 500–750 mg twice daily can also be used with excellent results.

References

Glick M, Cleveland DB. Oral mucosal bacillary (epithelial) angiomatosis in a patient with AIDS associated with rapid alveolar bone loss: report of a case. *Oral Pathol Med* 1993;22:235–239.

Manders S. Bacillary angiomatosis. *Clin Dermatol* 1996;14: 245–249.

Maurin M, Raoult D. *Bartonella (Rochalimaea) quintana* infections. *Clin Microbiol Rev* 1996;9:289–305.

Behçet Disease

■ Definition

Behçet disease is a chronic multisystemic relapsing inflammatory disorder of uncertain cause and prognosis. It is classified among the systemic vasculitides.

■ Etiology

The etiology of Behçet disease remains unknown, however, there is ample evidence favoring multifactorial pathogenesis. Autoimmunity may be one of the factors. Recently it has been proposed that the tumor necrosis factor (TNF) may play a central role in the pathogenesis of this inflammatory process.

■ Main Clinical Features

The disease usually begins during the third decade of life and there are periods of remission and exacerbation. The main clinical features include oral lesions, genital ulcerations, skin and ocular lesions, and arthropathy. The pathergy test is positive in approximately 50–60% of the cases.

Oral Lesions

Aphthous ulcers (minor, major, herpetiform or atypical ulcers) are the most common and occur early in the course of the disease

Genital Lesions

Genital ulcers, similar to aphthous ulcers, in the scrotum, penis, and vulva are common

Skin Lesions

Papules, pustules, nodules, erythema nodosum, folliculitis, necrotic angiitis, and ulcers are the most common skin lesions

Ocular Lesions

Conjunctivitis, iritis with hypopyon, uveitis, and retinal vasculitis (which may occasionally lead to blindness)

Other Features

Seronegative mono-polyarthritis, epididymitis, venous thrombosis, arterial aneurysms, glomerulonephritis, pulmonary vasculitis, pericarditis, endocarditis, neurological disorders, and others

■ Diagnosis

The diagnosis of Behçet disease is based almost exclusively on the history and the clinical features, since there are no pathognomonic laboratory tests.

■ Differential Diagnosis

- Aphthous ulcers
- FAPA syndrome
- Herpes simplex infection
- Erythema multiforme
- Stevens–Johnson syndrome
- Reiter syndrome
- Pyostomatitis vegetans
- Pemphigus
- Cicatricial pemphigoid
- Systemic lupus erythematosus
- Ulcerative colitis
- Crohn disease
- Rheumatoid diseases
- Lung sarcoidosis

■ Treatment

Basic Guidelines

- Accurate diagnosis is the most important step for successful therapy.
- A team of specialists should be involved in the treatment of Behçet disease, including a stomatologist, an ophthalmologist, a dermatologist, a rheumatologist, a gastroenterologist, and others. The treatment is adapted to the individual patient based on their clinical signs and symptoms.
- Both topical and systemic treatments are used. Mild forms of the disease respond well

to topical treatment, while in severe and multisystemic forms systemic treatment is required.

- The treatment of severe forms must be undertaken by the specialists.

Suggested Therapies

Systemic Treatment

Corticosteroids

Systemic oral corticosteroids, usually prednisone, are the drugs of choice for the treatment of Behçet disease. The initial dose varies from 30 mg/day to 80 mg/day or more depending on the severity of the disease and organ involved. After the disease has been controlled the dose is tapered gradually to 5–10 mg/day for long periods of time. Corticosteroids may be used either alone or in combination with azathioprine or other immunosuppressives.

Immunosuppressive Drugs

Azathioprine 50–100 mg/day appears to be effective, particularly for ocular and oral lesions. Cyclosporine 2–3 mg/kg day, cyclophosphamide 1–2 mg/kg day, chlorambucil 0.1 mg/kg day have also been used, in particular, for the treatment of ocular lesions. These drugs are used with or without corticosteroids.

Other Drugs

Colchicine 0.5–2 mg/day, and dapsone 100 mg/day can be used to treat particular oral and cutaneous lesions. Thalidomide 50–200 mg/day seems to be effective for oral lesions. Colchicine and thalidomide are absolutely contraindicated during pregnancy. Pentoxifylline 800 mg/day has recently been used, particularly for the treatment of oral, cutaneous, and ocular lesions. Nonsteroidal anti-inflammatory drugs are helpful in cases where there is joint involvement.

Topical Treatment

Painful oral aphthous ulcers require topical treatment alone or usually in association with systemic treatment.

Topical treatment is aimed at a) elimination of pain and discomfort, b) shortening of the duration of lesions, and c) avoidance of recurrence. Topical corticosteroids in the form of 0.1% triamcinolone acetonide, or 0.05% clobetasol in an oral adhesive base (Orabase), or fluocinonide gel applied to the ulcer three to six times a day, are the mainstay of topical therapy. Inhaled corticosteroids have also been used for ulcers in the soft palate and posterior vestibule.

Topical anesthetics such as 5% lidocaine (Xylocaine) ointment or viscous gel or diphenhydramine hydrochloride (Benadryl elixir) reduce the pain for a short time only. Recently, 5% amlexanox (Aphthasol) oral paste or 3% diclofenac in 2.5% hyaluronan has been shown to reduce the pain and shorten the duration of the ulcers. Topical tetracycline mouthwashes or application of tetracycline compresses have been used with partial success. Topical 5% 5-aminosalicylic acid or silver nitrate stick application may provide relief from pain and shorten the duration of the ulcers.

Genital ulcers and skin lesions can be treated topically with corticosteroids and antimicrobial ointments or creams. Local treatment of ocular lesions must be undertaken by an ophthalmologist.

Alternative Therapies

Interferon alpha, mycophenolate mofetil, tacrolimus, sulfasalazine, and anticoagulants have been suggested as alternative treatments in severe and resistant cases. Recently, rebamipide (a gastroprotective drug) has been recommended as a long-term adjunctive treatment for recurrent oral aphthous ulcers in patients with Behçet disease. Anti-TNF therapy has also been used with success.

References

Binnie WH, Curro FA, Khandwala A, Van Inwegan RG. Amlexanox oral paste: a novel treatment that accelerates the healing of aphthous ulcers. *Compend Contin Educ Dent* 1997;118:1116–1118, 1120–1122.

Collier PM, Neill SM, Copeman PW. Topical 5-aminosalicylic acid: A treatment for aphthous ulcers. *Br J Dermatol* 1992;126:185–188.

De Tran QH, Guay E, Chartier S, Tousignant J. Tacrolimus in dermatology. *J Cutan Med Surg* 2001;5:329–335.

Goker B, Goker H. Current therapy for Behçet's disease. *Am J Ther* 2002;9:465–470.

Matsuda T, Ohno S, Hirohata Y, et al. Efficacy of rebamipide as adjunctive therapy in the treatment of recurrent oral aphthous ulcers in patients with Behçet's disease: a randomized, double-blind, placebo-controlled study. *Drugs R D* 2003;4:19–28.

Sfikakis PP. Behçet's disease: A new target for anti-tumour necrosis factor treatment. *Ann Rheum Dis* 2002;61(suppl 2):51–53.

Sharquie KE, Najim RA, Abu-Raghif AR. Dapsone in Behçet's disease: A double-blind, placebo-controlled, crossover study. *J Dermatol* 2002;29:267–279.

Shek LP, Lim DL. Thalidomide in Behçet's disease. *Biomed Pharmacother* 2002;56:31–35.

Stratigos A, Laskaris G, Laskaris J. Behçet's disease. *Semin Neurol* 1992;12:346–357.

Benign Tumors

■ Definition

Benign tumors are common in the oral cavity and originate from the epithelium, connective tissue, nerves, vessels, muscles, and other oral tissues.

■ Etiology

The etiology of the great majority of oral benign tumors is unknown. Some of them are reactive or developmental.

■ Classification

- Papilloma
- Fibroma
- Peripheral ossifying fibroma
- Osteoma
- Chondroma
- Lipoma
- Myxoma
- Neurofibroma
- Schwannoma
- Traumatic neuroma
- Leiomyoma
- Rhabdomyoma
- Verruciform xanthoma
- Granular cell tumor
- Granular cell tumor of the newborn
- Fibrous histiocytoma
- Hemangioma
- Lymphangioma
- Papillary syringadenoma
- Melanotic nevi
- Melanotic neuroectodermal tumor of infancy
- Pleomorphic adenoma
- Myoepithelioma
- Other salivary gland adenomas
- Pyogenic granuloma
- Peripheral giant cell granuloma

■ Main Clinical Features

- Firm or soft, raised, usually well defined, asymptomatic swelling
- Tumor may be sessile or pedunculated
- Size varies from 0.5 cm to several centimeters
- Color may be normal, yellowish, white, red, bluish, or black

■ Diagnosis

The clinical diagnosis should be confirmed by biopsy and histopathologic examination.

■ Differential Diagnosis

The differential diagnosis includes all benign tumors, soft tissue cysts, and malignant neoplasms.

■ Treatment

- Conservative surgical excision is the treatment of choice for all benign tumors.
- Electrosurgery, laser surgery, or cryotherapy can also be used as alternative methods of treatment for some benign tumors.
- Details of the surgical procedures and techniques are beyond the scope of this book.

References

Laskaris G. *Color Atlas of Oral Diseases*, 3rd edition. Thieme Verlag: Stuttgart, 2003.
Neville BW, Damm DD, Allen CM, Bouquot JE. *Oral and Maxillofacial Pathology*, 2nd edition. WB Saunders Co, Philadelphia, 2002.
Sailer HF, Pajarola GF. *Oral Surgery for the General Dentist*. Thieme Verlag: Stuttgart, 1999.

Buccal Cellulitis

■ Definition

Cellulitis is a relatively common infectious process of the dermis and subcutaneous tissues.

■ Etiology

Staphylococcus aureus and *S. pyogenes* are the most common causative organisms. Cellulitis in children can also be caused by group A streptococci and *Haemophilus influenzae.*

■ Main Clinical Features

- Systemic symptoms such as fever, chills, and malaise
- Diffuse, painful, firm, ill defined erythematous swelling that feels warm
- Vesicles, bullae, pustules, and tissue necrosis may occur in cases of severe infection
- Regional lymph node enlargement may occur

■ Diagnosis

The diagnosis is usually based on the clinical criteria. Blood culture, needle aspiration, and rarely, a biopsy can be done.

■ Differential Diagnosis

- Trauma
- Insect bites
- Erysipelas
- Venous thrombosis
- Superficial thrombophlebitis
- Panniculitis
- Sweet syndrome
- Vasculitis
- Acute parotitis
- Other inflammatory disorders

■ Treatment

Basic Guidelines

- In the majority of cases treatment should be directed against *S. pyogenes* and *S. aureus.*
- Culture and antibiotic sensitivity tests should be done in severe and antibiotic-resistant cases.
- Treatment should be implemented rapidly to avoid complications.
- Hospitalization and parenteral antibiotics should be reserved for children with severe illness.

Suggested Therapies

- Empiric initial treatment can be instituted with one of the following drugs: oral cloxacillin 250–500 mg every 6 hours; oral dicloxacillin 125–500 mg every 6 hours; oral flucloxacillin 250–500 mg every 6 hours; or oral amoxicillin 250–500 mg every 8 hours. Mild cases require 10 days treatment.
- Oral ciprofloxacin 250–750 mg twice daily alone or in combination with metronidazole 250–500 mg every 8 hours may also be used, in particular in more severe cases.

Alternative Therapies

Oral levofloxacin 200–750 mg daily or twice daily is recommended for patients with complicated cellulitis. Recently, linezolid in a dose of 400 mg every 12 hours has been recommended.

References

Bouvet A. Cellulitis and necrotizing fasciitis: microbiology and pathogenesis. *Ann Dermatol Venereol* 2001;128: 382–389.

Lewis R. Soft tissue infections. *World J Surg* 1998;22:146–151.

Matson KL, Miller SE. Tooth discoloration after treatment with linezolid. *Pharmacotherapy* 2003;23:682–685.

Sachs M. Cutaneous cellulitis. *Arch Dermatol* 1991;124: 493–500.

Taylor CO, Carter JB. Buccal cellulitis in an infant due to ampicillin-resistant *Haemophilus influenzae. J Oral Maxillofac Surg* 1986;44:234–239.

Bullous Pemphigoid

■ Definition

Bullous pemphigoid is a chronic bullous disease primarily affecting the skin and, less often, the mucous membranes. It commonly affects middle-aged and elderly individuals.

■ Etiology

Bullous pemphigoid is an autoimmune disease. Bullous pemphigoid antigens 180 (BP180) and 230 (BP230) have been identified as the target antigens, and autoantibodies to these antigens are pathogenetically critical.

■ Main Clinical Features

The oral mucosa is affected in about 30–40% of cases and usually follows skin involvement. Bullous pemphigoid may rarely be associated with internal malignant disease.

Oral Mucosa

- Localized or scattered bullae that rupture leaving persistent painful erosions
- Palatal and buccal mucosa, tongue, lips, and gingiva are more frequently affected
- Rarely the oral lesions are the first manifestations

Other Mucosae

- Conjunctiva, esophagus, vagina, and anus are affected less frequently

Skin

- Nonspecific generalized rash and tense bullae, isolated or in clusters, that rupture leaving erosions without a tendency to extend peripherally
- Nikolsky sign is negative

■ Diagnosis

The clinical diagnosis should be confirmed by histopathologic examination and direct and indirect immunofluorescence. Circulating anti-basement membrane antibodies can be found in the sera of about 70–80% of patients.

■ Differential Diagnosis

- Pemphigus
- Cicatricial pemphigoid
- Linear IgA disease
- Pemphigoid gestationis
- Epidermolysis bullosa acquisita
- Dermatitis herpetiformis
- Erythema multiforme
- Stevens–Johnson syndrome
- Bullous and erosive lichen planus
- Bullous systemic lupus erythematosus

■ Treatment

Basic Guidelines

- Systemic and topical treatments should be used in the management of bullous pemphigoid depending on the severity of the disease. The age of the patient and the presence of other diseases should be also taken into consideration.
- Severe and moderate disease with oral lesions usually need systemic corticosteroids alone or in combination with immunosuppressives or dapsone.
- Localized mild disease with oral or skin lesions alone may initially be treated with local corticosteroids.
- The side effects of systemic corticosteroid therapy must always be taken into account and the patients should be regularly examined both clinically and by laboratory testing for this possibility.
- Patients with oral lesions should avoid mechanical injuries and should be advised to maintain good oral hygiene.

Suggested Therapies

Systemic Treatment

Oral Corticosteroids

Oral corticosteroids are the mainstay of therapy for bullous pemphigoid. The majority of patients with generalized disease usually respond well to 40–80 mg/day of prednisone or prednisolone. It usually takes 2–3 weeks to stop new bullae formation and for old lesions to heal. Once the disease is controlled, the dose of the corticosteroid is tapered slowly over months and finally the drug is withdrawn. Recurrences are not unusual.

Immunosuppressive Drugs

Azathioprine 50–100 mg/day appears to be effective and it is the most commonly used corticosteroid-sparing agent for bullous pemphigoid. Cyclophosphamide 100–200 mg/day or cyclosporine 5–8 mg/kg per day also appears to be effective. Recently, mycophenolate mofetil 2 g/day has been used either in combination with corticosteroids or as monotherapy in the treatment of bullous pemphigoid with considerable success.

Dapsone/Sulfapyridine

Dapsone 50–100 mg/day or sulfapyridine 2–4 g/day might be effective in some cases (10–15%) of bullous pemphigoid, in particular in younger patients or patients with localized oral lesions.

Topical Treatment

Localized oral or skin lesions may be successfully treated with topical corticosteroids alone. This treatment may be given either in the form of oral paste or ointment, or in the form of an intralesional injection.

Alternative Therapies

- Tetracycline/niacinamide: Tetracycline 1.5–2.0 g/day alone or in combination with niacinamide 1.5 g/day are useful, particularly for controlling limited disease.
- Plasmapheresis: This can be used as an adjuvant to corticosteroids in selected severe cases of bullous pemphigoid.
- Future therapies of bullous pemphigoid might be directed toward the induction of compensating BP180 and BP230 isoforms.
- Topical use of tacrolimus in an adhesive paste form may also be useful for localized oral lesions.

References

Böhm M, Beissert S, Schwarz T, et al. Bullous pemphigoid treated with mycophenolate mofetil. *Lancet* 1997, 349:541.

Grundmann-Kollmann M, Kaskel P, Leiter U, et al. Treatment of pemphigus vulgaris and bullous pemphigoid with mycophenolate mofetil monotherapy. *Arch Dermatol* 1999;135:724–725.

Joly P, Roujeau JC, Benichou J, et al. A comparison of oral and topical corticosteroids in patients with bullous pemphigoid. *N Engl J Med* 2002;346:321–327.

Korman NJ. New immunomodulating drugs in autoimmune blistering diseases. *Dermatol Clin* 2001;19:637–648.

Liu Z, Diaz LA. Bullous pemphigoid: End of the century overview. *J Dermatol* 2001;28:647–650.

Stern RS. Bullous pemphigoid therapy—think globally, act locally. *N Engl J Med* 2002;346:364–367.

Wojnarowska F, Kirtschig G, Khumalo N. Treatment of subepithelial immunobullous diseases. *Clin Dermatol* 2001; 19:768–777.

Burkitt Lymphoma

Definition

Burkitt lymphoma is a high-grade malignancy of B-lymphocyte origin that usually affects the jaws.

Etiology

Epstein–Barr virus has been implicated in the pathogenesis of Burkitt's lymphoma.

Classification

There are three types of Burkitt lymphoma: a) African, b) endemic, and c) American or sporadic.

Main Clinical Features

- Pain, tenderness, paresthesia, bone destruction, and tooth mobility and loss are common symptoms and signs
- A large ulcerating or nonulcerating soft tissue mass may also be present in the oral mucosa and gingiva
- The maxilla is more frequently affected than the mandible
- Usually affects children 2–12 years of age

Diagnosis

The clinical diagnosis should be confirmed by a biopsy and histopathologic examination.

Differential Diagnosis

- Non-Hodgkin lymphoma
- Osteosarcoma
- Chondrosarcoma
- Ewing's sarcoma
- Multiple myeloma
- Cherubism
- Central giant cell granuloma
- Odontogenic tumors

Treatment

- Chemotherapy—CHOP (cyclophosphamide, doxorubicin, vincristine, and prednisone) regimens or more complex chemotherapy—is the treatment of choice, either alone or in combination with radiotherapy and surgery. This regimen has improved the prognosis of Burkitt lymphoma.
- Radiation therapy is the second treatment choice, either alone or in combination with chemotherapy.
- Surgery can also be used for early localized lesions.

References

Hesseling PB, Broadhead R, Molyneux E, et al. Malawi pilot study of Burkitt lymphoma treatment. *Med Pediatr Oncol* 2003;41:532–540.

Levine AM. Challenges in the management of Burkitt's lymphoma. *Clin Lymphoma* 2002;3(suppl 1):S19–S25.

Philip T, Bergeron C. Burkitt's lymphoma: A model for pediatric oncology. *Arch Pediatr* 2000;7:924–926.

Shapira J, Peylan-Ramu N. Burkitt's lymphoma. *Oral Oncol* 1998;34:15–23.

Wang ES, Straus DJ, Teruya-Feldstein J, et al. Intensive chemotherapy with cyclophosphamide, doxorubicin, high-dose methotrexate-ifosfamide, etoposide, and high-dose cytarabine (CODOX-M/IVAC) for human immunodeficiency virus-associated Burkitt's lymphoma. *Cancer* 2003;98:1196–1205.

Weinthal JA, Goldman SC, Lenarsky C. Successful treatment of relapsed Burkitt's lymphoma using unrelated cord blood transplantation as consolidation therapy. *Bone Marrow Transplant* 2000;25:1311–1313.

Candidiasis

▣ Definition

Candidiasis is the most frequent fungal infection of the oral cavity.

▣ Etiology

Candida albicans is the most common candida species to cause oral candidiasis. Other species such as *C. glabrata, C. tropicalis, C. krusei, C. parapsilosis, C. dubliniensis* can cause infections though less frequently. *Candida* species are normally present on mucocutaneous body surfaces, and several local and systemic predisposing factors are necessary to develop infection with clinical symptoms and signs.

▣ Classification

Oral candidiasis is clinically classified as primary and secondary. Primary candidiasis includes several clinical forms such as pseudomembranous, erythematous, nodular, and *Candida*-associated lesions (angular cheilitis, median rhomboid glossitis, denture stomatitis). Secondary candidiasis includes chronic mucocutaneous and *Candida*-endocrinopathy syndrome. Systemic candidiasis is less common than superficial *Candida* infection, but it is an increasing problem in immunocompromised patients. Candidemia is now recognized as the fourth most important nosocomial bloodstream infection.

▣ Main Clinical Features

The oral mucosa is the most common site of superficial candidiasis. However, the vagina, glans penis, skin, and nails may also be involved.

Pseudomembranous (Thrush)

- The most common form of oral candidiasis, usually acute. It appears as creamy whitish spots or plaques, which usually can be detached. The lesions may be localized or generalized. Burning, dryness, loss of taste, and pharyngeal dysphagia are common symptoms

Erythematous

It appears as erythematous patches usually on the dorsum of the tongue and palate. This form is common in HIV-infected patients and in patients on antibiotics. Burning is a common symptom

Nodular

A chronic form of candidiasis that appears as white, firm, raised plaques that cannot be detached. The lesions are usually asymptomatic

Candida-Associated Lesions

Angular cheilitis: red, fissured crusts with or without erosions. Whitish spots or plaques may be present
Median rhomboid glossitis: reddish smooth or nodular surface on the midline of the dorsum of the tongue
Denture stomatitis: diffuse erythema and edema of the mucosa underneath a denture

Secondary Forms

Chronic mucocutaneous candidiasis: chronic oral lesions, skin and nail lesions as well. Classically the oral lesions are generalized
Candida-endocrinopathy syndrome: severe oral, skin, and nail lesions associated with endocrinopathies appear early in life from 4–6 years of age

▣ Diagnosis

The diagnosis of candidiasis is usually based on clinical criteria. Direct smear microscopic examination with potassium hydroxide and culture are helpful. Biopsy and histopathologic examination may also be useful in some cases.

▣ Differential Diagnosis

- Leukoplakia
- Hairy leukoplakia
- Lichen planus

- Lupus erythematosus
- Mucous patches of secondary syphilis
- White sponge nevus
- Uremic stomatitis
- Cinnamon contact stomatitis
- Chemical burns
- Traumatic lesions
- Furred tongue

Treatment

Basic Guidelines

- Elimination of systemic and/or local predisposing factors are important to avoid recurrences.
- Maintenance of high level of oral hygiene and reduction of the *Candida* reservoir in the mouth, esophagus, and genitalia.
- Accurate diagnosis of the clinical form of oral candidiasis is important.
- Topical or systemic therapy should be used depending on the form and severity of the disease.
- The majority of the available antifungal drugs target the synthesis of ergosterol, a constituent of the fungal cell membrane.

Suggested Therapies

Systemic Treatment

Systemic azoles are the drugs of choice. Itraconazole capsules 100 mg/day or fluconazole 100 mg/day for 1–2 weeks are usually effective for acute pseudomembranous candidiasis and *Candida*-associated lesions. The erythematous and nodular forms usually need therapy for 2–4 weeks. The secondary forms need long-term administration of the above drugs in a dose of 100–200 mg/day for 1–3 months.

Ketoconazole capsules 200 mg twice daily for 1–4 weeks, depending the form of the disease, may also be used. In patients with resistant *Candida* species, in neutropenic patients, or in patients with malignancies, transplants, and AIDS, itraconazole oral solution 2.5–5 mg/kg per day is indicated. Ketoconazole has significantly greater bioavailability than itraconazole and, in addition, has a topical effect; therefore it may convey additional benefits over other oral agents in the treatment of oral candidiasis. It must be remembered that successful systemic treatment of oral candidiasis often depends on correction or treatment of the predisposing factors.

The use of systemic azole derivatives can be impaired by interference with gastric pH, by interactions with other drugs such as rifampicin, acyclovir, cyclosporine, phenytoin, H_2-antagonists, terfenadine, astemizole, or by the emergence of resistant or less susceptible strains of *Candida*.

Clinicians should avoid systemic azoles in patients with severe liver disease and during pregnancy. The most frequent side effects of itraconazole and fluconazole are gastrointestinal symptoms (nausea, vomiting, diarrhea, epigastralgia) and rash.

Topical Treatment

Nystatin oral suspension four times a day or miconazole oral gel 5 ml four times a day for 1–2 weeks is indicated, particularly for oral acute pseudomembranous candidiasis in infants or children or for adults where systemic treatment is not indicated. Angular cheilitis (perlèche) is treated with topical antifungal ointments.

Future Therapies

Third generation triazoles (voriconazole, posaconazole, ravuconazole), echinocandins (main representative caspofungin) and the incorporation of nystatin into liposomes are being investigated as possible alternative treatments.

References

Davies A, Brailsford S, Broadley K, Beighton D. Resistance amongst yeasts isolated from the oral cavities of patients with advanced cancer. *Palliat Med* 2002;16:527–531.

Dismukes WE. Introduction to antifungal drugs. *Clin Infect Dis* 2000;30:653–657.

Ellepola ANB, Samaranayake LP. Antimycotic agents in oral candidosis: An overview: 2. Treatment of oral candidosis. *Dent Update* 2000;27:165–174.

Epstein JB, Gorsky M, Caldwell J. Fluconazole mouthrinses for oral candidiasis in postirradiation, transplant, and other patients. *Oral Surg Oral Med Oral Pathol Oral Radiol Endod* 2002;93:671–675.

Fratti RA, Belanger PH, Samati H. The effect of the new triazole, voriconazole (UK-109,496) on the interactions of *Candida albicans* and *Candida krusei* with endothelial cells. *J Chemother* 1998;10:7–16.

Goins RA, Ascher D, Waecker N, et al. Comparison of fluconazole and nystatin oral suspensions for treatment of oral candidiasis in infants. *Pediatr Infect Dis J* 2002;21:1165–1167.

Groll AH, Wood L, Roden M, et al. Safety, pharmacokinetics, and pharmacodynamics of cyclodextrin itraconazole in pediatric patients with oropharyngeal candidiasis. *Antimicrob Agents Chemother* 2002;46: 2554–2563.

Johnson LB, Kauffman CA. Voriconazole: A new triazole antifungal agent. *Clin Infect Dis* 2003;36:630–637.

Koks CHW, Meenhorst PL, Bult A, Beijnen JH. Itraconazole solution: Summary of pharmacokinetic features and review of activity in the treatment of fluconazole-resistant oral candidiasis in HIV-infected persons. *Pharmacol Res* 2002;46:195–201.

Koltin Y, Hitchock CA. Progress in the search for new triazole antifungal agents. *Curr Opin Chem Biol* 1997;1:176–182.

Tacconelli E, Bertagnolio S, Posteraro B, et al. Azole susceptibility patterns and genetic relationship among oral *Candida* strains isolated in the era of highly active antiretroviral therapy. *J Acquir Immune Defic Syndr* 2002;31:38–44.

Terrell CL. Antifungal agents. Part II. The azoles. *Mayo Clin Proc* 1999;74:78–100.

Villanueva A, Gotuzzo E, Arathoon EG, et al. A randomized double-blind study of caspofungin versus fluconazole for the treatment of esophageal candidiasis. *Am J Med* 2002;113:294–299.

Worthington HV, Clarkson JE. Prevention of oral mycositis and oral candidiasis for patients with cancer treated with chemotherapy: Cochrane systematic review. *J Dent Educ* 2002;66:903–911.

Cheilitis Glandularis

■ Definition

Cheilitis glandularis is a rare chronic inflammatory disorder of the lower lip characterized by hyperplasia of the minor salivary glands.

■ Etiology

The etiology of cheilitis glandularis is unknown.

■ Main Clinical Features

- Lip enlargement
- Typically, the orifices of the secretory ducts become dilatated and appear as numerous pinhead openings from which mucus or mucopurulent secretion may be expressed on pressure
- Crusting, erosions, and microabscesses may occur
- Characteristically, the lesions are limited to the lower lip

■ Diagnosis

The clinical diagnosis should be confirmed by a biopsy and histopathologic examination.

■ Differential Diagnosis

- Cheilitis granulomatosa
- Melkersson–Rosenthal syndrome
- Crohn disease
- Orofacial granulomatosis
- Sarcoidosis
- Tuberculosis
- Lymphedema
- Lymphangioma

■ Treatment

Basic Guidelines

- There is no causative treatment.
- The treatment is palliative.

Suggested Therapies

- Topical ointment or intralesional injection of corticosteroids may offer temporary and limited improvement.
- Systemic oral corticosteroids, e.g., prednisone 20–30 mg/day for 2–3 weeks, followed by tapering and stopping the drug in a month's time has also limited value as the disease recurs.
- Systemic antibiotics, e.g., minocycline 100–200 mg/day for 2–4 weeks, may temporarily improve the condition, particularly if an infection is present.
- Plastic surgery (vermilionectomy) for reconstruction of an enlarged lip is necessary for advanced severe cases.

References

Cohen DM, Green JG, Diekmann SL. Concurrent anomalies: Cheilitis glandularis and double lip: report of a case. *Oral Surg Oral Med Oral Pathol* 1988;66:397–399.

Leao JC, Ferreira AM, Martins S, et al. Cheilitis glandularis: An unusual presentation in a patient with HIV infection. *Oral Surg Oral Med Oral Pathol Oral Radiol Endod* 2003;95:142–144.

Stoopler ET, Carrasco L, Stanton DC, et al. Cheilitis glandularis: An unusual histopathologic presentation. *Oral Surg Oral Med Oral Pathol Oral Radiol Endod* 2003; 95:12–17.

Swerlick RA, Cooper PH. Cheilitis glandularis: A reevaluation. *J Am Acad Dermatol* 1984;10:466–472.

Venma S. Cheilitis glandularis: A rare entity. *Br J Dermatol* 2003;148:362.

Cheilitis Granulomatosa

▪ Definition

Cheilitis granulomatosa, or Miescher cheilitis, is an uncommon, chronic, noncaseating granulomatous inflammatory disorder.

▪ Etiology

The etiology of cheilitis granulomatosa is unknown, however, a cell-mediated hypersensitivity to foods, food additives, and flavoring agents may play a role in the development of the disease.

▪ Main Clinical Features

Cheilitis granulomatosa may occur as an isolated disorder or as part of other granulomatous diseases, e.g., Melkersson–Rosenthal syndrome, Crohn disease, and sarcoidosis.

- Painless, diffuse swelling of the upper or lower lip or both
- Small vesicles, erosions, and scaling may rarely develop
- Lesions may appear suddenly and have a chronic course with remissions and exacerbations
- Permanent enlargement of the lips may occur

▪ Diagnosis

The clinical diagnosis should be confirmed by a biopsy and histopathologic examination.

▪ Differential Diagnosis

- Cheilitis glandularis
- Melkersson–Rosenthal syndrome
- Crohn disease
- Sarcoidosis
- Orofacial granulomatosis
- Tuberculosis
- Angioedema
- Lymphedema
- Lymphangioma
- Foreign body reaction

▪ Treatment

Basic Guidelines

- Before treatment systemic granulomatous diseases should be excluded.
- Food additives, flavoring agents, some foods, and foreign materials should be ruled out as causative agents.

Suggested Therapies

- Intralesional corticosteroids such as triamcinolone acetonide or betamethasone dipropionate and sodium phosphate retard are recommended as initial therapy. A course of 3–6 intralesional injections may be used.
- Systemic corticosteroids, e.g., prednisone 30–40 mg/day for about 2–3 weeks and then gradually tapered over 1–3 months, may significantly improve the condition.
- Minocycline 100–200 mg/day for 3–6 months in combination with systemic corticosteroids is the best therapeutic regimen.
- Clofazimine, thalidomide, hydroxychloroquine, sulfasalazine, and dapsone have also been used as second-line treatments.
- Plastic surgery reconstruction is indicated in advanced, chronic cases with lip disfiguration.

References

Arbiser JL, Moschella SL. Clofazimine: A review of its medical uses and mechanisms of action. *J Am Acad Dermatol* 1995;32:241–247.

Rees TD. Orofacial granulomatosis and related conditions. *Periodontology* 2000 1999;21:145–157.

Ridder GJ, Fradis M, Lohle E. Cheilitis granulomatosa Miescher: Treatment with clofazimine and review of the literature. *Ann Otol Rhinol Laryngol* 2001;110:964–967.

Stein SL, Mancini AJ. Melkersson–Rosenthal syndrome in childhood: Successful management with combination steroid and minocycline therapy. *J Am Acad Dermatol* 1999;41:746–748.

Thomas P, Walchner M, Ghoreschi K, Rocken M. Successful treatment of granulomatous cheilitis with thalidomide. *Arch Dermatol* 2003;139:136–138.

Van der Waal RI, Suhulten EA, van der Meij EH, et al. Cheilitis granulomatosa: Overview of 13 patients with long-term follow-up results of management. *Int J Dermatol* 2002;41:225–229.

Veller FC, Catalano P, Peserico A. Minocycline in granulomatous cheilitis: Experience with 6 cases [letter]. *Dermatology* 1992;185:220.

Chemical Burns

▨ Definition

Red or red and white mucosal lesion resulting from contact to the oral mucosa with chemical agents.

▨ Etiology

Common culprits include phenol, trichloroacetic acid, eugenol, aspirin, iodine, alcohol, acrylic resin, sodium perborate, silver nitrate, sodium hypochlorite, paraformaldehyde, chlorine compounds, and agricultural chemical agents.

▨ Main Clinical Features

- Improper use of chemical agents in the oral cavity may result in inflammation, ulceration, and coagulative necrosis of the epithelium (white, desquamating lesion)
- Lesions may be painful or not, depending on the severity of the burn
- Chemical burns are usually localized to the area of contact with the chemical agent
- Severity depends on the extent and duration of the contact as well as the concentration and quantity of the compound

▨ Diagnosis

The diagnosis is based on the history and the clinical features.

▨ Differential Diagnosis

- Vesiculobullous diseases
- Candidiasis
- Mechanical trauma
- Thermal burns
- Erythroplakia
- Squamous cell carcinoma

▨ Treatment

Basic Guidelines

- Avoid spices, hard and hot foods.
- Mild chemical burns such as those due to alcohol, iodine, sodium hypochlorite, or sodium perborate usually heal within a week.
- More severe burns such as those caused by chlorine, trichloracetic acid, and other more caustic agents usually take up to 2 weeks to heal.

Suggested Therapies

- Usually none needed.
- In severe persistent cases oral corticosteroids in low doses for a short time, e.g., prednisone 10–15 mg/day for 3–5 days, dramatically improve the symptoms.

References

Fantasia JE, Damm DD. White mucosa. Chemical burn. *Gen Dent* 2001;49:265, 324.

Flaitz CM. Chemical burn of the labial mucosa and gingiva. *Am J Dent* 2001;14:259–260.

Milano M. Oral electrical and thermal burns in children: Review and report of case. *J Dent Child* 1999;66:116–119.

Mordjikian E. Severe microstomia due to burn by caustic soda. *Burns* 2002;28:802–805.

Nahlieli O, Eliav E, Shapira Y, Baruchin AM. Central palatal burns associated with the eating of microwaved pizzas. *Burns* 1999;25:465–466.

Treharne LJ, Kay AR. The initial management of acute burns. *J R Arm Med Corps* 2001;147:198–205.

Chronic Ulcerative Stomatitis

■ Definition

Chronic ulcerative stomatitis is a newly described, rare oral disease with characteristic immunofluorescent findings.

■ Etiology

Chronic ulcerative stomatitis is an autoimmune disease with characteristic specific antinuclear antibodies directed against stratified epithelium.

■ Main Clinical Features

The disease involves, almost exclusively, the oral mucosa and has a chronic course with recurrences.

Oral Mucosa

- Gingival lesions usually appear in the form of *desquamative gingivitis*
- Oral mucosal lesions (buccal mucosa and tongue) appear as painful erosions or ulcers, usually associated with white reticular lesions identical to those seen in oral lichen planus

■ Diagnosis

The clinical diagnosis should be confirmed by histopathologic examination and particularly by direct and indirect immunofluorescent tests.

■ Differential Diagnosis

- Lichen planus
- Discoid lupus erythematosus
- Cicatricial pemphigoid
- Linear IgA disease
- Bullous pemphigoid
- Epidermolysis bullosa acquisita
- Pemphigus
- Oral psoriasis
- Idiopathic form of desquamative gingivitis

■ Treatment

Basic Guidelines

- Patients with gingival involvement should avoid the use of hard toothbrushes or any mechanical friction.
- Systemic or local treatment may be used depending on the severity of the disease.
- Recurrence may occur after cessation of treatment.

Suggested Therapies

Systemic Treatment

Hydroxychloroquine

Hydroxychloroquine (Plaquenil) 200–300 mg/day is the treatment of choice for chronic ulcerative stomatitis. The lesions usually respond to treatment in 1–2 weeks and may disappear in about a month.

Oral Corticosteroids

Prednisone or prednisolone 20–40 mg/day reduce the symptoms and lesions heal in approximately 2–4 weeks. Then the dose is tapered slowly by 20% every 2 weeks. Topical corticosteroids may be used to maintain the results.

Topical Treatment

The use of 0.1% triamcinolone acetonide in an oral adhesive base (Orabase), fluocinolone acetonide in an oral paste or 0.05% clobetasol propionate gel either alone (in mild lesions) or after control of severe lesions by systemic treatment is usually effective, particularly in cases of desquamative gingivitis. Intralesional injections of triamcinolone acetonide for extragingival lesions is also helpful.

References

Chorzelski TP, Olszewska M, Jarzabek-Chorzelska M, Jablonska S. Is chronic ulcerative stomatitis an entity? Clinical and immunological findings in 18 cases. *Eur J Dermatol* 1998;8:261–265.

Jaremko WM, Beutner EH, Kumar V, et al. Chronic ulcerative stomatitis associated with a specific immunologic marker. *J Am Acad Dermatol* 1990;22:215–220.

Lewis JE, Beutner EH, Rostami R, Chorzelski TP. Chronic ulcerative stomatitis with stratified epithelium-specific antinuclear antibodies. *Int J Dermatol* 1996;35:272–275.

Worle B, Wollenberg A, Schaller M, et al. Chronic ulcerative stomatitis. *Br J Dermatol* 1997;137:262–265.

Cicatricial Pemphigoid

■ Definition

Cicatricial pemphigoid or mucous membrane pemphigoid is a chronic, recurrent, autoimmune blistering disease that primarily affects mucous membranes and rarely the skin. Cicatricial pemphigoid represents a heterogeneous group of diseases with respect to disease severity, clinical site of involvement, and the isotype of the associated autoantibodies.

■ Etiology

Cicatricial pemphigoid is an autoimmune condition. Hemidesmosome and lamina lucida proteins, bullous pemphigoid antigen 180 (BP180), laminins 5, β_4 integrin, and type VII collagen have been identified as the target antigens in cicatricial pemphigoid.

■ Main Clinical Features

The oral mucosa is almost always affected, followed by other mucosae (ocular, nose, pharynx, larynx, esophagus, genitalia, anus) and rarely the skin (5–10%).

Oral Mucosa

Erythema and bullae that rupture leaving painful erosions. The lesions usually recur, persist for a long time, and occasionally lead to atrophy or scarring. The soft palate, buccal mucosa, and the gingiva are more frequently affected in the form of *desquamative gingivitis*. The oral lesions may be the only manifestations of the disease

Ocular Mucosa

Conjunctivitis, symblepharon, trichiasis, dryness, and opacity of the cornea—occasionally leading to blindness

Other Mucosae

Bullae that rupture leaving erosions that may lead to scarring

Skin

Bullae that usually develop on the scalp, face, and neck and may heal with or without scarring

■ Diagnosis

The clinical diagnosis should be confirmed by histopathologic examination and direct and indirect immunofluorescence tests.

■ Differential Diagnosis

- Lichen planus (erosive and bullous forms)
- Bullous pemphigoid
- Linear IgA disease
- Chronic ulcerative stomatitis
- Epidermolysis bullosa acquisita
- Pemphigus
- Dermatitis herpetiformis
- Erythema multiforme
- Herpetic stomatitis
- Plasma cell stomatitis

■ Treatment

Basic Guidelines

- Systemic or topical treatment is for the management of cicatricial pemphigoid depending on the severity of the disease and the organs involved.
- Patients with oral lesions should avoid mechanical injuries from hard and rough foods, toothbrushes, broken teeth, fillings with rough margins, and dentures. Dentists must use dental instruments gently.
- Systemic or topical corticosteroid administration is the mainstay of treatment. Immunosuppressive drugs should also be used as adjuvant therapy in severe and resistant cases.
- One of the most serious morbidities of cicatricial pemphigoid is ocular involvement. These patients must be managed in consultation with an expert ophthalmologist.

Suggested Therapies

Systemic Treatment

Oral Corticosteroids

Oral corticosteroids (prednisone or prednisolone) are the cornerstone of therapy for cicatricial pemphigoid. The initial dose varies from 30 mg/day to 60 mg/day depending on the severity of the disease. It usually takes 2–3 weeks to stop new bullae formation and for old ones to heal. The dose is subsequently tapered by 20% every 2–3 weeks until the dose of 10 mg/day is reached. This dose is subsequently maintained on alternate days and reduced by 5 mg every 2 weeks until it is completely stopped. Recurrence of oral lesions is not uncommon and may be treated with local corticosteroids or low doses of systemic corticosteroids.

Immunosuppressants

Corticosteroid-sparing immunosuppressants are usually required only in severe cases that present with ocular, laryngeal, or esophageal involvement because of the increased risk for blindness and scar formation. Azathioprine 100 mg/day and cyclophosphamide 100–200 mg/day are most frequently used. Mycophenolate mofetil 2 g/day may also be used in some cases.

Dapsone

50–100 mg/day is beneficial in mild to moderate diseases, particularly for patients with oral lesions alone.

Topical Treatment

Localized, mild, oral lesions or recurrences may be treated with topical corticosteroids alone; 0.1% triamcinolone acetonide in an oral adhesive base (Orabase), or 0.5% fluocinonide gel, or 0.05% clobetasol propionate gel applied to the lesions two to three times a day for 2–6 months or more is particularly effective for gingival lesions (desquamative gingivitis). Recently, 0.05% clobetasol mouthwash in aqueous solution has been shown to be effective for localized oral lesions. Intralesional injection of triamcinolone acetonide retard or betamethasone dipropionate and sodium phosphate retard may be beneficial for localized resistant oral lesions. Topical cyclosporine is another feasible therapy for patients with oral lesions.

Alternative Therapies

Recently, new immunomodulators for topical use, with anti-inflammatory action, such as tacrolimus and 0.1% pimecrolimus ointment, have been used with promising results in the treatment of oral lesions of autoimmune diseases. Combination therapy with tetracyclines (minocycline or doxycycline) 1–2 g/day and nicotinamide 1–2 g/day may be effective.

References

Chan LS, Ahmed AR, Anhalt GJ, et al. The first international consensus on mucous membrane pemphigoid: Definition, diagnostic criteria, pathogenic factors, medical treatment and prognostic indicators. *Arch Dermatol* 2002;138:370–379.

Eisen D, Ellis CN, Woorhees JJ. Topical cyclosporine for oral bullous disorders. *J Am Acad Dermatol* 1990;23:936–937.

Gonzalez-Moles MA, Morales P, Rodriguez-Archilla A, et al. Treatment of severe chronic oral erosive lesions with clobetasol propionate in aqueous solution. *Oral Surg Oral Med Oral Pathol Oral Radiol Endod* 2002;93:264–270.

Korman NJ. New immunomodulating drugs in autoimmune blistering diseases. *Dermatol Clin* 2001;19:637–648.

Reiche L, Wojnarowska F, Mallon E. Combination therapy with nicotinamide and tetracyclines for cicatricial pemphigoid: Further support for efficacy. *Clin Exp Dermatol* 1998;23:254–257.

Schmidt E, Skrobek C, Kromminga A, et al. Cicatricial pemphigoid: IgA and IgG autoantibodies target epitopes on both intra- and extracellular domains of bullous pemphigoid antigen 180. *Br J Dermatol* 2001;145:778–783.

Wojnarowska F, Kirtschig G, Khumalo N. Treatment of subepidermal immunobullous diseases. *Clin Dermatol* 2001;19:768–777.

Cinnamon Contact Stomatitis

■ Definition

Cinnamon contact stomatitis is a relatively common reaction of the oral mucosa secondary to the chronic use of substances with artificial cinnamon flavoring.

■ Etiology

The stomatitis is a result of use of cinnamon products such as chewing gum, candy, toothpaste, dental floss, oral solutions etc.

■ Main Clinical Features

- Redness of the oral mucosa usually associated with desquamation and erosions or ulcerations
- Hyperkeratotic white plaques are common
- Burning and pain are common symptoms
- Buccal mucosa and the lateral borders of the tongue are more frequently affected
- Exfoliative cheilitis and perioral dermatitis may occur

■ Diagnosis

The diagnosis is based on the history and the clinical features.

■ Differential Diagnosis

- Amalgam contact stomatitis
- Chronic biting
- Leukoedema
- Lichen planus
- Leukoplakia
- Candidiasis
- Hairy leukoplakia
- Plasma cell stomatitis
- Uremic stomatitis
- Lupus erythematosus
- Epithelial peeling

■ Treatment

Basic Guidelines

- High level of oral hygiene should be maintained.
- Change or avoid any product which contains cinnamon.
- Avoid antibacterial mouthwashes as these worsen the symptoms.
- If the cinnamon products are reused usually the signs and symptoms soon recur.

Suggested Therapies

- Discontinuation of any cinnamon product improves the condition and the signs and symptoms disappear in approximately 2 weeks time.
- In cases of severe and extended erosions, corticosteroids in the form of topical ointment or low doses of oral prednisone, e.g., 10–15 mg/day for 1 week, help the lesions to heal soon.
- Topical rinses with chamomile four to five times daily improve the symptoms.

References

Allen CM, Blozis GG. Oral mucosal reactions to cinnamon-flavored chewing gum. *JADA* 1988;116:664–667.

Le Sueur BW, Yiannias JA. Contact stomatitis. *Dermatol Clin* 2003;21:105–114.

Miller R, Gould A, Berstein M. Cinnamon-induced stomatitis venenata. *Oral Surg Oral Med Oral Pathol* 1992;73:708–716.

Samio EL, Kanerva L. Contact allergens in toothpastes and a review of their hypersensitivity. *Contact Dermatitis* 1995;33:100–105.

Coccidioidomycosis

▨ Definition

Coccidioidomycosis is a chronic systemic mycosis, endemic in the USA, Central America, and South America.

▨ Etiology

Coccidioides immitis, a dimorphic fungus, is the causative organism.

▨ Main Clinical Features

There are five clinical forms of the disease: a) acute pulmonary, b) chronic pulmonary, c) disseminated focal, d) disseminated widespread, and e) meningitis. Oral lesions develop in disseminated infection, which commonly occurs in patients with AIDS or in immunocompromised patients.

Oral Lesions

These present as vegetating ulcers with irregular peripheries. The palate, tongue, and gingiva are more frequently affected.

Disseminated Widespread Form

Fever, malaise, anorexia, cough, chest pain, weight loss, and lymphadenopathy are common signs and symptoms. With time, lesions develop in the bone, joints, skin, subcutaneous tissues, meninges, and other sites.

▨ Diagnosis

Smear, culture, and biopsy are very useful diagnostic tools. Serologic tests are also helpful.

▨ Differential Diagnosis

- Paracoccidioidomycosis
- Other systemic mycoses
- Squamous cell carcinoma
- Tuberculosis
- Syphilis
- Non-Hodgkin lymphoma
- Leishmaniasis

▨ Treatment

Basic Guidelines

These are as for the other systemic mycoses.

Suggested Therapies

- Itraconazole 100–400 mg/day for 12 months or more is useful in the treatment of coccidioidomycosis.
- Ketoconazole 200–400 mg/day for 12 months or more has resulted in improvement in patients with lung, skin, bone, and joint lesions.
- Fluconazole 100–300 mg/day may be useful.
- Amphotericin B 0.5–0.7 mg/kg per day for about 12–14 weeks is recommended in severe disease, particularly in patients with meningitis.

Future Therapies

Voriconazole has been shown to have in-vitro activity against *C. immitis*.

References

Diaz M, Puente R, de Hoyos LA, Cruz S. Itraconazole in the treatment of coccidioidomycosis. *Chest* 1991;100:682–684.

Drutz DJ. Amphotericin B in the treatment of coccidioidomycosis. *Drugs* 1983;26:337–341.

Ghannoum MA, Kuhn DM. Voriconazole: Better changes for patients with invasive mycoses. *Eur J Med Res* 2002;7:242–256.

Graybill JR, Stevens DA, Galgiani JN, et al. Itraconazole treatment of coccidioidomycosis. *Am J Med* 1990;89:282–290.

Condyloma Acuminatum

▣ Definition

Condyloma acuminatum or anogenital wart is a common benign viral-induced lesion.

▣ Etiology

Types 6 and 11 human papilloma virus (HPV) are the main causative organisms of the disease.

▣ Main Clinical Features

The lesions are usually found on the anogenital area and rarely in the oral mucosa. Oral condyloma acuminatum may result from autoinoculation from anogenital lesions or during oro–genital contact.

Oral Lesions

- Single or multiple small sessile or pedunculated painless nodules with cauliflower surface
- The lesions have normal or whitish color
- Lip and buccal mucosa, gingiva, and palate are the sites of predilection

Anogenital Lesions

- Discrete or multiple, sessile or pedunculated, exophytic, small nodules with cauliflower-like appearance
- Lesions may have whitish or brown color
- Size varies from 1–5 mm to several cm in diameter

▣ Diagnosis

Biopsy and histopathologic examination confirms the diagnosis. In-situ hybridization may be useful in difficult cases.

▣ Differential Diagnosis

- Verruca vulgaris
- Papilloma
- Verruciform xanthoma
- Focal epithelial hyperplasia
- Sialadenoma papilliferum
- Molluscum contagiosum
- Focal dermal hypoplasia syndrome
- Early verrucous carcinoma

▣ Treatment

Basic Guidelines

- There is no specific antiviral therapy.
- The treatment of oral lesions should be followed by the treatment of anogenital lesions, if present.
- The oral lesions rarely recur.
- The treatment of anogenital warts must be provided by a dermatologist.

Suggested Therapies

- Conservative surgical excision of oral condyloma acuminatum is the treatment of choice—the procedure is quick and safe.
- Electrosurgery, cryotherapy, or CO_2 laser may be used as alternative therapeutic measures for the treatment of oral lesions.
- Anogenital lesions are treated with a) cytotoxic agents, b) physical procedures, and c) immunomodulatory agents.

Future Therapies

Prophylactic vaccination.

References

Coremans G, Margaritis V, Snoeck R, et al. Topical cidofovir (HPMPC) is an effective adjuvant to surgical treatment of anogenital condylomata acuminata. *Dis Colon Rectum* 2003;46:1103–1108.

Garland SM. Imiquimod. *Curr Opin Infect Dis* 2003;16:85–89.

Gunter J. Genital and perianal warts: New treatment opportunities for human papillomavirus infection. *Am J Obstet Gynecol* 2003;189(suppl 3):S3–11.

Smith KJ, Hamza S, Skelton H. The imidazoquinolines and their place in the therapy of cutaneous disease. *Expert Opin Pharmacother* 2003;4:1105–1119.

Stanley MA. Progress in prophylactic and therapeutic vaccines for human papillomavirus infection. *Expert Rev Vaccines* 2003;2:381–389.

Tsambaos D, Georgiou S, Monastirli A, et al. Treatment of condylomata acuminata with oral isotretinoin. *J Urol* 1997;158:1810–1812.

Contact Cheilitis

■ Definition

Contact cheilitis is an acute or chronic inflammatory disorder of the lips resulting from contact with various allergens or irritants.

■ Etiology

The most common causes are lipsticks, lip salves, toothpastes, mouthwashes, foods, etc.

■ Main Clinical Features

- Mild edema and erythema, followed by scaling and fissures or plaques
- Dryness and a burning sensation are common
- Rarely blisters may develop
- Angular cheilitis is usually present

■ Diagnosis

A careful medical history is important to determine the probable cause. Patch testing is the standard to confirm the diagnosis.

■ Differential Diagnosis

- Exfoliative cheilitis
- Plasma cell cheilitis
- Actinic cheilitis
- Herpes simplex
- Lip licking cheilitis

■ Treatment

Basic Guidelines

- It is important to attempt to identify the causative allergen before treatment.
- Once the allergens have been identified, the patient should avoid them.
- The physician should note down information on all of the probable allergens.

Suggested Therapies

- Systemic oral corticosteroids, e.g., prednisone 20–30 mg/day for 1–2 weeks and then tapering the dose and finally stopping it in 2–3 weeks is the first-line treatment, particularly in severe cases.
- Topical corticosteroids, e.g., a low potency ointment for about 2–3 weeks may control the disease, particularly in mild cases. However, the clinician should be aware of the possibility of allergy to local corticosteroid therapy. It should be suspected when the topical treatment fails to cure the condition or an exacerbation occurs after the use of corticosteroids.

References

Boffa MJ, Wilkinson SM, Beck HM. Screening for corticosteroid contact hypersensitivity. *Contact Dermatol* 1995;33:149–151.
Cohen DE, Brancaccio R. What is new in clinical research in contact dermatitis. *Dermatol Clin* 1997;15:137–148.
Freeman S, Stephens R. Cheilitis: Analysis of 75 cases referred to a contact dermatitis clinic. *Am J Contact Dermatol* 1999;10:198–200.
Holmes G, Freeman S. Cheilitis caused by contact urticaria to mind flavoured toothpaste. *Australas J Dermatol* 2001;42:43–45.
Riera Ras P, Ras Monleon RM. Management of contact cheilitis in primary care. *Aten Primaria* 1998;15:53–58.

Crohn Disease

■ Definition

Crohn disease is a chronic granulomatous disease of the entire gastrointestinal tract.

■ Etiology

The exact etiology of Crohn disease is unknown. However, an immune mechanism probably participates in the pathogenesis.

■ Main Clinical Features

Oral manifestations occur in 10–30% of patients with Crohn disease. Occasionally the oral lesions precede the intestinal involvement.

Oral Lesions

- Granulomatous lip swelling
- Edematous, firm painless nodules with or without ulcerations
- Mucosal tags
- Multiple nodules resulting in a "cobblestone" pattern of the buccal mucosa
- Gingival swelling
- Angular cheilitis
- Erythema and scaling of perioral skin
- Aphthous-like lesions
- Pyostomatitis vegetans
- Regional lymphadenopathy

Abdominal Lesions

- Abdominal pain
- Nausea and diarrhea with or without blood
- Vomiting
- Rectal bleeding
- Low-grade fever
- Weight loss and malnutrition

Others

- Anemia
- Short stature and decreased growth
- Arthritis and spondylitis
- Uveitis

■ Diagnosis

The diagnosis should be confirmed by a biopsy and histopathologic examination.

■ Differential Diagnosis

- Cheilitis granulomatosa
- Melkersson–Rosenthal syndrome
- Sarcoidosis
- Orofacial granulomatosis
- Tuberculosis
- Foreign body reaction

■ Treatment

Systemic Treatment

A variety of drugs—corticosteroids, sulfasalazine and mesalamine, immunosuppressive agents, and antibiotics—and nutritional therapy are employed for the treatment of Crohn disease. The presenting form of the disease, which may be one of three broad categories, i.e., inflammatory, fistulizing, or fibrostenotic, determines the type of therapy. Active inflammatory disease, whether in the small bowel or colon, is best treated with oral 5-aminosalicylic acid (5-ASA) 3 g/day and/or antibiotics (metronidazole 1500 mg/day). If these agents are not sufficient to induce remission, corticosteroid treatment (e.g., prednisone 40–60 mg) is warranted to arrest the inflammation rapidly; it is then gradually tapered. Many patients need the minimum dose of 7.5–10 mg corticosteroid to keep the disease in remission. Infliximab is very effective in controlling the symptoms of acute and chronic active disease when other treatments fail. In severe fistulizing disease, metronidazole, ciprofloxacin, and azathioprine have been successfully used. Infliximab (chimeric antibody against TNF) has proved to be highly effective in treating fistulas and is the treatment of choice when other treatments fail. Obstruction simply because of fibrostenotic Crohn disease usually resolves spontaneously in 1–2 days with simple conservative and supportive management (i.v. fluids, nil by mouth, i.v. steroids). Probiotics, human anti-

TNF, thalidomide, mycophenolate mofetil, tacrolimus, and interleukin 10/11 are promising treatment alternatives under research.

Topical Treatment

- Intralesional corticosteroid injection two to four times every 2 weeks may be used as adjuvant therapy for oral lesions.
- Surgical excision of mucosal tags and folds.

References

Castiglione F, Rispo A, Di Girolamo E, et al. Antibiotic treatment of small bowel bacterial overgrowth in patients with Crohn's disease. *Aliment Pharmacol Ther* 2003;18:1107–1112.

Kalmar JR. Crohn's disease: Orofacial considerations and disease pathogenesis. *Periodontol 2000* 1994;6;101–115.

Sandborn WJ. Optimizing anti-tumor necrosis factor strategies in inflammatory bowel disease. *Curr Gastroenterol Rep* 2003;5:501–505.

Sawczenko A, Lynn R, Sandhu BK. Variations in initial assessment and management of inflammatory bowel disease across Great Britain and Ireland. *Arch Dis Child* 2003;88:990–994.

Steinhart A, Ewe K, Griffiths A, et al. Corticosteroids for maintenance of remission in Crohn's disease. *Cochrane Database Syst Rev* 2003;4:CD000301.

Cryptococcosis

■ Definition

Cryptococcosis is a rare, life-threatening systemic fungal disease.

■ Etiology

The causative organism is *Cryptococcus neoformans* and two varieties have been identified: *C. neoformans* var. *neoformans* and *C. neoformans* var. *gattii.* Predisposing conditions include HIV infection, Hodgkin disease, chronic lymphocytic leukemia, organ transplantation, diabetes mellitus, and immunosuppressive treatment.

■ Main Clinical Features

There are two main types of cryptococcosis: a) pulmonary, which is the common, and b) disseminated. The oral mucosa is rarely affected in disseminated cryptococcosis.

Oral Lesions

The oral lesions present as chronic ulcers with an abnormal border and vegetating surface which is tender on palpation. The tongue, palate, gingiva, and a post tooth extraction socket are the most common sites of involvement.

Pulmonary Cryptococcosis

The most common signs and symptoms are cough, malaise, dyspnea, hemoptysis, chest pain, pleurisy, low-grade fever, night sweats, and weight loss. Approximately 30% of patients with pulmonary cryptococcosis are asymptomatic.

Disseminated

Cryptococcal central nervous system infection usually presents as subacute or chronic meningoencephalitis. Involvement of the kidneys, prostate, liver, spleen, adrenals, and lymph nodes may occur. Multiple papules or nodules may occur on the skin either as part of the disseminated disease or as solitary localized lesions.

■ Diagnosis

Biopsy and histopathologic examination, positive culture, and cryptococcal serum and cerebrospinal fluid antigen detection.

■ Differential Diagnosis

- Histoplasmosis
- Aspergillosis
- Mucormycosis
- Other systemic mycoses
- Squamous cell carcinoma
- Tuberculosis
- Eosinophilic ulcer
- Non-Hodgkin lymphoma
- Salivary gland malignancies
- Leishmaniasis

■ Treatment

Basic Guidelines

- Treatment of oral cryptococcosis is part of the systemic treatment of the disseminated form of the disease and should be undertaken only by the specialist.
- Early diagnosis and treatment of oral lesions are important for the course of the disease.
- Treatment of acute cryptococcal disease has dramatically improved survival over the past 15–20 years.
- Control and treatment of predisposing conditions are necessary for successful outcome.

Suggested Therapies

- Amphotericin B 0.5–1 mg/kg per day or more with or without flucytosine 150 mg/kg per day is regarded as the best initial therapy for patients with meningitis or more severe illness. Amphotericin B is administered for 2 weeks, followed by oral fluconazole 400 mg/day for an additional 6–8 weeks. This therapeutic regimen has been shown to be quite effective.
- Fluconazole 20–30 mg/kg per day, alone or in combination with flucytosine, is highly effica-

cious in the treatment and prevention of meningoencephalitis. Fluconazole 200–300 mg/day plus flucytosine seems to be efficacious for mild cases. Fluconazole 200 mg/day may also be used as maintenance therapy decreasing the relapse rate.

- Itraconazole 200–400 mg/day alone or in combination with flucytosine 150–200 mg/kg per day can be used as alternative treatment for cryptococcosis; in particular, this regimen is recommended as maintenance therapy to prevent relapse.

Future Therapies

The third generations triazoles, e.g., posaconazole and voriconazole, seem to be effective against *C. neoformans*.

References

Apisarnthanarak A, Powderly WG. Treatment of acute cryptococcal disease. *Expert Opin Pharmacother* 2001; 2:1259–1268.

Barchiesi F, Schimizzi AM, Caselli F, et al. Activity of the new antifungal triazole, posaconazole, against *Cryptococcus neoformans*. *J Antimicrob Chemother* 2001;48: 769–773.

Ghannoum MA, Kuhn Dm. Voriconazole: better changes for patients with invasive mycoses. *Eur J Med Res* 2002;7:242–256.

Hossain MA, Mukherjee PK, Reyes G, et al. Effects of fluconazole singly and in combination with 5-fluorocytosine or amphotericin B in the treatment of cryptococcal meningoencephalitis in an intracranial murine model. *J Chemother* 2002;14:351–360.

Kotwani RN, Gokhale PC, Bodhe PV, et al. Safety and efficacy of liposomal amphotericin B in patients with cryptococcal meningitis. *J Assoc Phys India* 2001;49:1086–1090.

Neuville S, Dromer F, Morin O, et al. Primary cutaneous cryptococcosis: A distinct clinical entity. *Clin Infect Dis* 2003;36:337–347.

Virgili A, Zampino MR, Mantovani L. Fungal skin infections in organ transplant recipients. *Am J Clin Dermatol* 2002;3:19–35.

Cyclic Neutropenia

Definition

Cyclic neutropenia is a rare hematologic disorder characterized by a regular cyclic reduction in the number of neutrophils.

Etiology

Cyclic neutropenia is an autosomal dominant trait with variable expression.

Main Clinical Features

The reduction in the number of neutrophils occurs regularly at 21-day intervals and generally lasts for 1–3 days. The disease usually manifests during infancy or childhood.

Oral Manifestations

- Painful oral ulcerations covered by a whitish membrane and surrounded by an erythematous halo
- Size of the ulcers varies from a few millimeters to 1 cm
- Gingivitis is common; periodontitis is rare
- Lips, buccal mucosa, tongue, and gingiva are more frequently affected

Other Manifestations

- Low-grade fever, malaise, headache, dysphagia, cervical lymphadenopathy, and arthralgias may occur
- Gastrointestinal ulcerations and skin infections are also common
- Symptoms and signs of cyclic neutropenia seem to diminish over time

Diagnosis

The clinical diagnosis should be confirmed by repeated complete blood counts, demonstrating the periodic reduction in the number of white blood cells.

Differential Diagnosis

- Aphthous ulcers
- Congenital neutropenia
- Agranulocytosis
- Aplastic anemia
- Leukemia
- Syphilis

Treatment

Basic Guidelines

- A high level of oral hygiene should be maintained with regular dental check-ups.
- Patients should avoid mechanical trauma during mastication and toothbrushing.
- Local application of antibiotic in periodontal pockets may be used as an auxiliary treatment, especially during neutropenic periods.
- Prophylactic systemic antibiotics should be avoided.
- Systemic treatment must be provided by a specialist.

Suggested Therapies

Topical Treatment

- Topical ointment of 0.1% triamcinolone acetonide in Orabase, or clobetasol gel two to four times daily reduce the pain and help the ulcers to heal sooner.
- 0.1% Chlorhexidine gluconate mouthwashes two to four times daily may be used to prevent local infection of the ulcers.
- 1% Povidone iodine solution and local antibiotic application may be helpful to improve the gingival condition.

Systemic Treatment

- Systemic oral corticosteroids, e.g., prednisone 10–20 mg/day during the acute phase improves the symptoms and signs.
- GM-CSF several times weekly may improve the neutrophil count; rhG-CSF is effective in shortening the recovery period in neutropenic patients.

- Systemic antibiotics should be given only if a systemic infection occurs.
- Splenectomy is an alternative treatment for severe, persistent cases.

References

Crawford J. Once-per-cycle pegfilgrastim (Neulasta) for the management of chemotherapy-induced neutropenia. *Semin Oncol* 2003;30(4 suppl 13):24–30.

Nakai Y, Ishihara C, Ogata S, Shimono T. Oral manifestations of cyclic neutropenia in a Japanese child: Case report with a 5-year follow-up. *Pediatr Dent* 2003;25:383–388.

Okada M, Kobayashi M, Hino T, et al. Clinical periodontal findings and microflora profiles in children with chronic neutropenia under supervised oral hygiene. *J Periodontol* 2001;72:945–952.

Pernu HE, Pajari UH, Lanning M. The importance of regular dental treatment in patients with cyclic neutropenia: Follow-up of 2 cases. *J Periodontol* 1996;67:454–459.

Cysts

Definition

The oral soft tissue cysts are a heterogeneous group of oral lesions.

Etiology

Most oral soft tissue cysts are developmental in origin, but mechanical trauma may be the cause of some.

Classification

- Mucocele
- Ranula
- Gingival cyst of the newborn
- Gingival cyst of the adult
- Eruption cyst
- Lymphoepithelial cyst
- Dermoid cyst
- Nasolabial cyst
- Palatine papilla cyst
- Thyroglossal cyst

Main Clinical Features

- Usually painless, occasionally fluctuant, soft tissue swelling is the common clinical finding for all cysts
- Color varies from normal to bluish or yellow
- Size varies from 0.5 cm to several centimeters
- Some cysts are common and others are rare

Diagnosis

The clinical diagnosis should be confirmed by histopathologic examination.

Differential Diagnosis

The differential diagnosis includes the various types of soft tissue cyst, benign tumor, and oral abscess.

Treatment

- Excision biopsy or conservative surgical excision or marsupialization (e.g., ranula) is the treatment of choice for all soft tissue cysts.
- Details of the surgical procedures and techniques are beyond of the scope of this book.

References

Baurmash HD. Mucoceles and ranulas. *J Oral Maxillofac Surg* 2003;61:369–378.

Binnie WH. Periodontal cysts and epulides. *Periodontol 2000* 1999;21:16–32.

Fuchshuber S, Grevers G, Issing WJ. Dermoid cyst of the floor of the mouth: A case report. *Eur Arch Otorhinolaryngol* 2002;259:60–62.

Giunta JL. Gingival cysts in the adult. *J Periodontol* 2002;73:827–831.

Laskaris G. *Color Atlas of Oral Diseases*, 3rd edition. Thieme Verlag: Stuttgart, 2003.

Manor Y, Buchner A, Peleg M, Taicher S. Lingual cyst with respiratory epithelium: An entity of debatable histogenesis. *J Oral Maxillofac Surg* 1999;57:124–127.

McGuff HS, Alderson GL, Jones AC. Oral and maxillofacial pathology case of the mouth. Gingival cyst of the adult. *Tex Dent J* 2003;120:108–112.

Norman JE, Head K. Ranula: This term is probably one of the oldest in surgery, and its etymology is not very obvious. *Br J Oral Maxillofac Surg* 2002;40:455–456.

Sailer HF, Pajarola GF. *Oral Surgery for the General Dentist*. Thieme Verlag: Stuttgart, 1999.

Tagagi S, Mizukawa N, Kimura T, Asaumi JI. Treatment of a plunging ranula with fenestration and continuous pressure. *Br J Oral Maxillofac Surg* 2003;41:410–413.

Dental Amalgam Contact Stomatitis

■ Definition

Dental amalgam contact stomatitis is a relatively common adverse toxic or hypersensitivity reaction of the oral mucosa to amalgam fillings.

■ Etiology

The offending agent is usually mercury and rarely other metals (zinc, copper, silver).

■ Main Clinical Features

- Redness and irregular white striae with or without erosions similar to those seen in oral lichen planus (lichenoid reaction)
- Burning and mild pain are common symptoms
- Characteristically, the lesions are confined to the area of the oral mucosa in contact with the amalgam
- Lesions most commonly develop in the buccal mucosa and the lateral borders of the tongue

■ Diagnosis

The diagnosis is usually based on the clinical features. Biopsy and histopathologic examination and a skin patch test for amalgam and inorganic mercury may also be done to aid the diagnosis.

■ Differential Diagnosis

- Lichen planus
- Lichenoid reactions due to drugs
- Allergic reactions to other dental materials
- Cinnamon contact stomatitis
- Discoid lupus erythematosus
- Candidiasis
- Plasma cell stomatitis

■ Treatment

Basic Guidelines

- A high level of oral hygiene should be maintained with removal of any accumulated plaque.
- Smooth and polish the dental amalgam fillings before any other treatment.
- Avoid antibacterial mouthwashes as they increase the symptoms.

Suggested Therapies

- Amalgam fillings should be removed and replaced with composite resin fillings or other materials in all patients with symptomatic lesions. Usually the lesions disappear in 2–4 weeks.
- Systemic oral corticosteroid in low doses, e. g., prednisone 10–20 mg/day for 1–2 weeks, are very helpful for severe lesions with extensive erosions. This regimen should be followed along with the replacement of the amalgam fillings.

References

Axell T. Hypersensitivity of the oral mucosa: Clinics and pathology. *Acta Odontol Scand* 2001;59:315–319.

Dunsche A, Kastel I, Terheyden H, et al. Oral lichenoid reactions associated with amalgam: Improvement after amalgam removal. *Br J Dermatol* 2003;148:70–76.

Garhammer P, Schmalz G, Hiller KA, et al. Patients with local adverse effects from dental alloys: frequency, complaints, symptoms, allergy. *Clin Oral Invest* 2001;5:240–249.

Little MC, Watson RE, Pemberton MN, et al. Activation of oral keratinocytes by mercuric chloride: relevance to dental amalgam-induced oral lichenoid reactions. *Br J Dermatol* 2001;144:1024–1032.

Lygre GB, Gjerdet NR, Gronningsaeter AG, Bjorkman L. Reporting on adverse reactions to dental materials–intraoral observations at a clinical follow-up. *Comm Dent Oral Epidemiol* 2003;31:200–206.

Denture Stomatitis

■ Definition

Denture stomatitis is a relatively common disorder usually confined to the palatal mucosa beneath the maxillary denture.

■ Etiology

The etiology of denture stomatitis is multifactorial. Poor fit and continuous wear of dentures for long periods of time, food debris, and *Candida albicans* are the most common etiologic factors.

■ Main Clinical Features

- Mucosa beneath the denture is red and edematous, with or without white spots (*Candida* hyphae)
- Papillary projections may develop in chronic cases
- Lesions are usually asymptomatic

■ Diagnosis

The diagnosis is based on the clinical criteria.

■ Differential Diagnosis

- Erythematous candidiasis
- Allergic contact stomatitis due to acrylic resin
- Acanthosis nigricans
- Systemic mycoses

■ Treatment

Basic Guidelines

- A high level of oral hygiene should be maintained with regular cleaning of the denture.
- Patients should be advised to remove their dentures at night.
- Reassure the patient that the lesion is innocent.
- In severe cases a new denture will be necessary.

Suggested Therapies

- The appropriate therapeutic modalities include improvement in denture fit, good oral hygiene, and topical application of nystatin or clotrimazole.
- In cases with severe *C. albicans* infection systemic itraconazole 100 mg/day or fluconazole 100 mg/day for 1–2 weeks is recommended.
- In cases with multiple papillary projections removal by electrosurgery and construction of a new denture are recommended.

References

Barbeau J, Seguin J, Goulet JP, et al. Reassessing the presence of *Candida albicans* in denture-related stomatitis. *Oral Surg Oral Med Oral Pathol Oral Radiol Endod* 2003;95:51–59.

Kazazoglu E, Arikan A. Oral hygiene habits, denture cleanliness, presence of yeasts and stomatitis in elderly people. *J Oral Rehabil* 2002;29:300–304.

Piloquet P, Daniel A, Giumelli B. Immunohistochemical localization of type IV collage and laminin (alpha 1) in denture stomatitis. J Oral Pathol Med 2001;30:98–103.

Vogel CW. Serotype distribution and secretory acid proteinase activity of *Candida albicans* isolated from the oral mucosa of patients with denture stomatitis. Oral Microbiol Immunol 1999;14:183–189.

Dermatitis Herpetiformis

Definition

Dermatitis herpetiformis or Duhring–Brocq disease is a rare, chronic, pruritic papulovesicular disease.

Etiology

Dermatitis herpetiformis is probably an autoimmune disease. Granular deposition of IgA and C_3 in the papillary dermis and along the basement membrane zone is diagnostic and a common finding in dermatitis herpetiformis. Although the target antigen is unknown, epidermal and tissue transglutaminase seems to be the dominant autoantigen both in the intestine and the skin.

Main Clinical Features

Dermatitis herpetiformis is a cutaneous manifestation of celiac disease and affects approximately 25% of patients with celiac disease. The oral mucosa is involved approximately in 5–10% and usually follows the skin eruption.

Oral Mucosa

The oral manifestations include localized, whitish maculopapular lesions, erythema and bullae that soon rupture leaving painful erosions. The buccal mucosa, lips, tongue, and palate are more frequently affected.

Skin

The cutaneous lesions appear as erythematous papules or plaques associated with burning and pruritus as well as small vesicles that coalesce in groups in a herpes-like pattern. The rash has a symmetrical distribution on the extensor surfaces of the elbows, proximal forearms, buttocks, posterior neck, back, and face. The disease has a prolonged course with periods of remission and exacerbation.

Diagnosis

The clinical diagnosis should be confirmed by histopathologic examination and direct and indirect immunofluorescence tests.

Differential Diagnosis

- Bullous pemphigoid
- Cicatricial pemphigoid
- Linear IgA disease
- Epidermolysis bullosa acquisita
- Pemphigus
- Prurigo
- Eczema

Treatment

Basic Guidelines

- A gluten-free diet is essential in the treatment of dermatitis herpetiformis, but drugs are usually needed in newly diagnosed disease to alleviate symptoms.
- Oral disease is usually secondary to skin lesions and may be treated either topically or systemically.
- All patients should be referred to a gastroenterologist and a dietician.

Suggested Therapies

Systemic Treatment

Dapsone

Oral dapsone is the mainstay of treatment for dermatitis herpetiformis. The starting dose is 100 mg/day. When the disease is controlled, usually in 2 weeks, the dose is slowly tapered to a minimal dose of 50 mg twice weekly for 2–3 months. If the disease is not controlled with 100 mg/day after 2 weeks, the dose should be increased to 200 mg/day. The side effects of dapsone must always be borne in mind.

Sulfapyridine

Oral sulfapyridine is the second-line drug for the treatment of dermatitis herpetiformis, particularly for those patients who are unable to tolerate dapsone. The initial dose is 1–2 g/day; it should be taken for at least 2 weeks and then the dose should be modified according to the response. Side effects include nausea, depression, lethargy, erythema multiforme, hemolytic anemia, and agranulocytosis.

Sulfamethoxypyridazine

Oral sulfamethoxypyridazine 0.5–1 g/day is an alternative therapeutic agent that may control the disease.

Gluten-Free Diet

A gluten-free diet is essential and usually improves both the enteropathy and dermatitis herpetiformis. It should be implemented along with the drug treatment. However, the patients should be highly motivated because gluten is ubiquitous and the diet should be followed for 1–2 years to control the disease. A gluten-free diet has also been found to reduce the incidence of lymphoma in patients with dermatitis herpetiformis. We recommend that patients receive advice regarding gluten-free diets from an expert dietician.

Topical Treatment

Topical corticosteroids may help in the healing of localized oral and skin lesions.

Alternative Therapies

Systemic corticosteroids, azathioprine, and a combination of heparin, tetracycline, and nicotinamide have been used where classic therapy has failed.

References

Collin P, Reunala T. Recognition and management of the cutaneous manifestations of celiac disease: A guide for dermatologists. *Am J Clin Dermatol* 2003;4:13–20.

Lewis H, Reunala T, Garioch J, et al. Protective effect of gluten-free diet against development of lymphoma in dermatitis herpetiformis. *Br J Dermatol* 1996;135:363–367.

Paniker U, Levine N. Dapsone and sulfapyridine. *Dermatol Clin* 2001;19:79–86.

Reunala TL. Dermatitis herpetiformis. *Clin Dermatol* 2001;19:728–736.

Shah SA, Ormerod AD. Dermatitis herpetiformis effectively treated with heparin, tetracycline and nicotinamide. *Clin Exp Dermatol* 2000;25:204–205.

Wojnarowska F, Kirtschig G, Khumalo N. Treatment of subepidermal immunobullous diseases. *Clin Dermatol* 2001;19:768–777.

Dermatomyositis

Definition

Dermatomyositis is a chronic systemic disorder characterized by inflammation of the skin and muscles.

Etiology

Dermatomyositis is an autoimmune disease.

Main Clinical Features

The oral cavity is not commonly affected. There is an increased risk of malignancy in patients with dermatomyositis.

Oral Lesions

The most frequent lesions are redness of the oral mucosa, painful edema, and ulcers.

Skin Lesions

A characteristic violaceous "heliotrope" rash of the upper eyelids is often present. Gottron's sign and papules over the knuckles and other joints are common. Telangiectasia and erythema of the proximal nail fords and poikilodermatous changes in sun-exposed areas are seen. Subcutaneous calcinosis may also be present.

Muscle Lesions

Progressive proximal muscle weakness is a typical sign. Pain and tenderness of affected muscles, Raynaud's phenomenon and joint symptoms may occur. Polymyositis occurs in association with Sjögren's syndrome, scleroderma, and systemic lupus erythematosus.

Diagnosis

The clinical diagnosis should be confirmed by histopathologic examination of skin and muscle biopsy. Serum muscle enzyme levels, especially aldolase and creatine phosphokinase, are useful aids to the diagnosis. Electromyography is also helpful.

Differential Diagnosis

- Systemic lupus erythematosus
- Stomatitis due to drugs
- Angioedema
- Scleroderma
- Lichen planus
- Polymorphous light eruption

Treatment

Basic Guidelines

- The oral lesions should be treated in collaboration with the dermatologist.
- The treatment should be adjusted according to the clinical variant and the course of the disease and should be provided by specialists.

Suggested Therapies

Corticosteroids

Systemic corticosteroids are used—prednisolone or prednisone, 40–60 mg/day, which is a suitable initial dose. Clinical control is usually achieved within 4–6 weeks, after which the dose is gradually tapered. Long-term steroid therapy, 10 mg/day or every other day, is often necessary to prevent recurrence.

Immunosuppressive Drugs

Cyclophosphamide 1–2 mg/kg per day, azathioprine 1–2 mg/kg per day, methotrexate 15–25 mg/week, and cyclosporine 3–5 mg/kg per day are effective second-line treatments. The newer immunosuppressive agents such as mycophenolate mofetil and tacrolimus are promising. Immunosuppressive drugs may be used alone or in combination with corticosteroids.

Alternative and Future Therapies

These include intravenous immunoglobulin, plasmapheresis, hydroxychloroquine, dapsone, anti-TNF-alpha therapy, and topical tacrolimus for managing the skin lesions.

References

Callen JP. Dermatomyositis: Diagnosis, evaluation and management. *Minerva Med* 2002;93:157–167.

Choy EH, Isenberg DA. Treatment of dermatomyositis and polymyositis. *Rheumatology (Oxford)* 2002;41:7–13.

Cohen JB. Cutaneous involvement of dermatomyositis can respond to dapsone therapy. *Int J Dermatol* 2002;41: 182–184.

Mastaglia FL, Zilko PJ. Inflammatory myopathies: How to treat the difficult cases. *J Clin Neurosci* 2003;10:99–101.

Oddis CV. Cyclosporin A and intravenous immunoglobulin treatment in polymyositis-dermatomyositis. *Curr Rheumatol Rep* 2002;4:401–402.

Sontheimer RD. Dermatomyositis: An overview of recent progress with emphasis on dermatologic aspects. *Dermatol Clin* 2002;20:387–408.

Wakata N, Kurihara T, Saito E, Kinoshita M. Polymyositis and dermatomyositis associated with malignancy: A 30-year retrospective study. *Int J Dermatol* 2002;41: 729–734.

Drug-Induced Gingival Overgrowth

■ Definition

Drug-induced gingival overgrowth or gingival hyperplasia is a relatively common side effect leading to gingival enlargement.

■ Etiology

The most common drugs causing gingival hyperplasia are phenytoin sodium, cyclosporine, calcium-channel blockers, and oral contraceptives. The dose of the drug, duration of therapy, level of oral hygiene, and other local factors influence the development of the gingival enlargement.

■ Main Clinical Features

- Painless gingival enlargement. The gingiva are firm, lobulated, slightly red, without a tendency to bleed
- Gingiva may progressively cover the crowns of the teeth
- Enlargement may be localized but is more often generalized

■ Diagnosis

The diagnosis is based on the medical history and the clinical features.

■ Differential Diagnosis

- Gingival fibromatosis
- Gingivitis
- Gingival overgrowth due to mouth breathing
- Leukemia
- Scurvy
- Wegener granulomatosis
- Gingival non-Hodgkin lymphoma
- Granulomatous diseases
- Amyloidosis
- Acanthosis nigricans
- Hurler syndrome
- Zimmermann–Laband syndrome
- Ramon syndrome
- Cross syndrome

■ Treatment

Basic Guidelines

- A high level of oral hygiene (plaque control, scaling) is mandatory.
- Discontinue or replace the drug with another whenever possible. This should be done by a specialist.
- A follow-up program by the dentist is recommended as recurrences are common if use of the causative drug is mandatory.

Suggested Therapies

- Conservative gingivectomy is the treatment of choice. This must always be done in conjunction with a preventive plaque-control program.
- Antiseptic rinses such as chlorhexidine may be useful to control plaque formation.
- In cases of mild gingival overgrowth the discontinuation of the responsible drug may be the only treatment required.

References

Brunet L, Miranda J, Roset P, et al. Prevalence and risk of gingival enlargement in patients treated with anticonvulsant drugs. *Eur J Clin Invest* 2001;31:781–788.

Camargo PM, Melnick PR, Pirih FQ, et al. Treatment of drug-induced gingival enlargement: Aesthetic and functional considerations. *Periodontol 2000* 2001;27: 131–138.

Hall EE. Prevention and treatment considerations in patients with drug-induced gingival enlargement. *Curr Opin Periodontol* 1997;4:59–63.

Hernandez G, Arriba L, Lucas M, de Andres A. Reduction of severe gingival overgrowth in a kidney transplant patient by replacing cyclosporin A with tacrolimus. *J Periodontol* 2000;71:1630–1636.

Hood KA. Drug-induced gingival hyperplasia in transplant recipients. *Prog Transplant* 2002;12:17–21.

Majola MP, McFadyen ML, Connolly C, et al. Factors influencing phenytoin-induced gingival enlargement. *J Clin Periodontol* 2000;27:506–512.

Rees TD. Drugs and oral disorders. *Periodontol 2000* 1998;18:21–36.

Drug-Induced Oral Ulcerations

■ Definition

Drug-induced oral ulcerations are a common side effect of many categories of drug.

■ Etiology

In theory, all drugs are capable of inducing adverse effects, which can be toxic, idiosyncratic, or allergic. The most common drugs are in the following categories: antibiotics, immunosuppressives, cancer chemotherapeutic drugs, nonsteroidal anti-inflammatory agents, nicorandil, alendronate, D-penicillamine, hydroxyurea, and several others.

■ Main Clinical Features

The side effects may occur in isolation on the oral mucosa or in association with similar lesions on the other mucosae and the skin.

- Painful erosions or ulcerations covered with whitish pseudomembranes with irregular margins usually surrounded by an erythematous halo
- Erythema with burning sensation is also common
- Lesions may be single or multiple
- Any area of the mouth may be involved. However, lesions are more common on the tongue, buccal mucosa, palate, lips, and the gingiva
- Lesions may appear during or after administration of the drug
- Lesions may occasionally be dose related

■ Diagnosis

The diagnosis is based on the medical history and the clinical features. Biopsy may help to rule out other oral diseases.

■ Differential Diagnosis

- Oral ulceration due to other medications
- Erythema multiforme

- Erosive lichen planus
- Aphthous ulcer
- Cicatricial pemphigoid
- Bullous pemphigoid
- Pemphigus
- Linear IgA disease
- Epidermolysis bullosa acquisita
- Lupus erythematosus

■ Treatment

Basic Guidelines

- The oral physician and dentists should maintain a high level of suspicion to drug-reaction in cases of persistent oral ulceration.
- High level of oral hygiene is mandatory in any case.
- Before final diagnosis avoid any use of antimicrobial mouthwashes.

Suggested Therapies

- Prompt recognition and withdrawal of suspicious medication in collaboration with the patient's physician or dentist is essential.
- Topical 0.1 % triamcinolone acetonide in Orabase, or 0.05 % clobetasol propionate gel or 0.1 % tacrolimus ointment applied to the ulcer three to four times daily for about one week time are an effective means of controlling the signs and symptoms of drug-induced oral ulceration. The topical treatment is recommended only if the oral lesions are localized. Intralesional injection of corticosteroid may also be used for persistent localized ulcers.
- Systemic oral corticosteroids, e.g., prednisone 10–20 mg/day for one or two weeks, is very effective in cases with disseminated and persistent oral ulcerations.
- Vitamin B complex may also help faster healing of the ulcer.

References

Abdollahi M, Radfar M. A review of drug-induced oral ulcerations. *J Contemp Dent* Pract 2003;4:10–31.

Boulinguez S, Sommet A, Bedane C, et al. Oral nicorandil-induced lesions are not aphthous ulcers. *J Oral Pathol Med* 2003;32:482–485.

Cella D, Pulliam J, Fuchs H, et al. Evaluation of pain associated with oral mucositis during the acute period after administration of high-dose chemotherapy. *Cancer* 2003;98:406–412.

Jeal W, Barradell LB, McTavish D. Alendronate: a review of its pharmacological properties and therapeutic efficacy in postmenopausal osteoporosis. *Drugs* 1997;53:415–434.

Laskaris G, Satriano R. Drug-induced blistering oral lesions. *Clin Dermatol* 1993;11:545–550.

Macario-Barrel A, Tanasescu S, Courville P, et al. Mouth ulcers in patients receiving tacrolimus. *Ann Dermatol Venereol* 2001;128:1327–1329.

Madinier I, Berry N, Chichmanian RM. Drug-induced oral ulcerations. *Ann Med Intern (Paris)* 2000;151:248–254.

Rees TD. Drug and oral disorders. *Periodontology 2000* 1998;18:21–36.

Scully C, Azul AM, Crighton A, et al. Nicorandil can induce severe oral ulceration. *Oral Surg Oral Med Oral Pathol Oral Radiol Endod* 2001;91:189–193.

Taukumova LA, Mouravjoy YV, Gribakin SG. Mucocutaneous side effects in continuation of aurotherapy in patients with rheumatoid arthritis. *Adv Exp Med Biol* 1999;455:367–373.

Vassallo C, Passamonti F, Merante S, et al. Mucocutaneous changes during long-term therapy with hydroxyuria in chronic myeloid leukemia. *Clin Exp Dermatol* 2001;26:141–148.

Witkowski JA, Parish LC. Cutaneous reactions of antibacterial agents. *Skin Med* 2002;1:33–44.

Drug-Related Mucosal Pigmentation

Definition

Drug-related pigmentation is a relatively common pigmentation of the oral mucosa.

Etiology

It may be caused by medications such as antimalarial agents, chemotherapeutic agents, and some other medications.

Main Clinical Features

- Usually diffuse pigmentation of the oral mucosa
- Minocycline pigmentation: Linear band above the facial aspect of the attached gingivae
- Antimalarials: Blue-black discoloration of the hard palate as well as diffuse brown staining of the oral mucosa

Diagnosis

The diagnosis is based on the history and the clinical features. Biopsy and histological examination may occasionally be necessary.

Differential Diagnosis

- Racial pigmentation
- Heavy metal deposition
- Addison disease
- Peutz–Jeghers syndrome
- Von Recklinghausen disease
- Albright syndrome

Treatment

- No treatment is needed.
- Discontinuation of the culprit medication will result in the pigmented areas fading over time.

References

Birek C, Main JH. Two cases of oral pigmentation associated with quinidine therapy. *Oral Surg Oral Med Oral Pathol* 1988;66:59–61.

Cale AE, Freedman PD, Lumerman H. Pigmentation of the jawbones and teeth secondary to minocycline hydrochloride therapy. *J Periodontol* 1988;59:112–114.

Cockings JM, Savage NW. Minocycline and oral pigmentation. *Aust Dent J* 1998;43:14–16.

Kleinegger CL, Hammond HL, Finkelstein MW. Oral mucosal hyperpigmentation secondary to antimalarial drug therapy. *Oral Surg Oral Med Oral Pathol Oral Radiol Endod* 2000;90:189–194.

Siller GM, Tod MA, Savage NW. Minocycline-induced oral pigmentation. *J Am Acad Dermatol* 1994;30:350–354.

Dry Socket

Definition

Dry socket, or alveolar osteitis is a relatively uncommon complication that occurs after extraction of a tooth, usually the posterior mandibular teeth.

Etiology

The exact etiology of dry socket is not fully known. After extraction, poor clot formation results in disordered fibrinolysis and local release of kinins and other potent pain mediators. Predisposing factors are local tissue damage, presurgical local bacterial infection, and oral contraceptives.

Main Clinical Features

- Dirty-gray clot that does not fill the socket
- Bare bony socket
- Exposed alveolar bone
- Severe pain
- Malodorous breath
- Swelling
- Regional lymphadenopathy
- Signs and symptoms develop 2–4 days following extraction of the tooth and may last for 2–4 weeks if left untreated

Diagnosis

The diagnosis is based exclusively on the history and clinical features.

Differential Diagnosis

- Retained root tip
- Impacted foreign body
- Pericoronitis
- Osteosarcoma
- Chondrosarcoma
- Malignant histiocytoma
- Other oral malignancies

Treatment

Basic Guidelines

- A "gentle" technique is recommended during surgical tooth extraction procedures.
- Preexisting pericoronitis or local infections should be treated before tooth extraction.
- Preventive local or systemic antibiotics therapy are not recommended.

Suggested Therapies

Systemic Treatment

Systemic administration of corticosteroids in low doses (e.g., 10–20 mg/day of prednisone) for 3–4 days relieves the pain immediately and in my experience is the best method for relief of pain. Systemic administration of antibiotics such as metronidazole 250–500 mg three times daily or tetracycline 500 mg three times daily may be helpful but should always be given in association with corticosteroids.

Topical Treatment

Packing the socket with an eugenol-containing iodoform gauze may be helpful. The dressing should be changed every 24 hours for the first 2–3 days and every 2–3 days thereafter. Topical rinsing of the socket with oxygenating agents and/or other antiseptics, or topical antifibrinolytics or antibiotics has been done with partial success.

References

Adeyemo WL. Critical review of dry socket. *Int J Oral Maxillofac Surg* 2003;32:111.

Blum IR. Contemporary views on dry socket (alveolar osteitis): a clinical appraisal of standardization, aetiopathogenesis and management: a critical review. *Int J Oral Maxillofac Surg* 2002;31:309–317.

Delilbasi C, Saracoglu U, Keskin A. Effects of 0.2% chlorhexidine gluconate and amoxicillin plus clavulanic acid on the prevention of alveolar osteitis following mandibular third molar extraction. *Oral Surg Oral Med Oral Pathol Oral Radiol Endod* 2002;94:301–304.

Oginni FO, Fatusi OA, Alagbe AO. A clinical evaluation of dry socket in a Nigerian teaching hospital. *J Oral Maxillofac Surg* 2003;61:871–876.

Eosinophilic Ulcer

■ Definition

Eosinophilic ulcer or traumatic eosinophilic granuloma is a benign self-limiting inflammatory lesion unrelated to eosinophilic granuloma of Langerhans cell histiocytosis.

■ Etiology

The etiology is unknown, although trauma may be the causative factor.

■ Main Clinical Features

- Sudden-onset painful ulcer with an irregular surface covered with a whitish pseudomembrane
- Raised inflammatory and indurated border
- Ulcers may be single or multiple
- Tongue is the site of predilection followed by the lips, buccal mucosa, and gingiva

■ Diagnosis

The diagnosis is based on a biopsy and histopathologic examination.

■ Differential Diagnosis

- Traumatic ulcer
- Major aphthous ulcer
- Syphilitic ulcer
- Tuberculosis
- Necrotizing sialadenometaplasia
- Non-Hodgkin lymphoma
- Leukemia
- Wegener granulomatosis
- Malignant granuloma

■ Treatment

Basic Guidelines

- Before treatment a biopsy is always necessary to rule out malignancy.
- The lesion is usually self-limiting and heals in several weeks or months.
- The healing time can be shortened by local and/or systemic treatment, which is recommended.

Suggested Therapies

Systemic oral corticosteroids, e.g., prednisone 20–30 mg/day or betamethasone 2–3 mg/day for 1 week and then tapering the dose and stopping it in about 1–2 weeks is the treatment of choice because the lesions heal quickly.

References

El Mofty SK, Swanson PE, Wick MR, Miller HS. Eosinophilic ulcer of the oral mucosa. Report of 38 new cases with immunohistochemical observations. *Oral Surg Oral Med Oral Pathol* 1993;75:716–722.

Gao S, Wang Y, Liu N, et al. Eosinophilic ulcer of the oral mucosa: A clinicopathological analysis. *Chin J Dent Res* 2000;3:47–50.

Kiderman A, Torten R, Furst AL, Reinus K. Bilateral eosinophilic ulcers in an infant treated with propolis. *J Dermatol Treat* 2001;12:29–31.

Sklavounou A, Laskaris G. Eosinophilic ulcer of the oral mucosa. *Oral Surg Oral Med Oral Pathol* 1984;58:431–436.

Epidermolysis Bullosa Acquisita

■ Definition

Epidermolysis bullosa acquisita is a rare, chronic, subepidermal mechanobullous disease involving the skin and mucous membranes.

■ Etiology

Epidermolysis bullosa acquisita is an autoimmune disorder. Type VII collagen has been identified as the main target antigen.

■ Main Clinical Features

The clinical diagnostic criteria for epidermolysis bullosa acquisita include skin fragility and blistering that may be spontaneous but are often induced by trauma. The lesions heal with scarring and milia formation. There is also absence of personal or family history of blistering disease. The disease usually involves mucous membranes (50%).

Oral Mucosa

Localized and, rarely, widespread bullae and painful erosions, particularly in friction-related areas of the oral mucosa. Gingival involvement may be either in the form of *desquamative gingivitis* or as localized bullae that rupture, leaving painful erosions. Scarring may also occur

Other Mucosae

These include ocular, nasal, esophageal, laryngeal, genital, and anal. Conjunctival and corneal scarring may lead to synechiae and rarely blindness. Esophageal, laryngeal, and anal scarring may also result in severe functional problems

Skin

The skin lesions present with marked fragility as hemorrhagic bullae and erosions usually at the site of trauma. The lesions heal with scarring and milia. Atrophic areas, hyperpigmentation, alopecia, and nail dystrophy may occur. The dorsum of the hands and arms, feet, knees, and elbows are more frequently affected. Localized or generalized involvement may occur

■ Diagnosis

The clinical diagnosis should be confirmed by histopathologic examination and direct and indirect immunofluorescence tests.

■ Differential Diagnosis

- Cicatricial pemphigoid
- Linear IgA disease
- Bullous pemphigoid
- Genetic epidermolysis bullosa
- Pemphigus
- Chronic ulcerative stomatitis
- Angina bullosa hemorrhagica
- Systemic bullous lupus erythematosus
- Dermatitis herpetiformis
- Porphyria cutanea tarda

■ Treatment

Basic Guidelines

- The disease usually responds poorly to therapeutic measures that control other bullous diseases.
- Systemic or topical therapies should be used depending on the severity of the disease and the organ involved.
- Mechanical irritation should be avoided and the patient should be made aware of the necessary lifestyle modifications required.
- Patients with oral lesions should be advised to avoid very hard foods and to use toothbrushes gently. Dentists should use dental instruments with caution in patients with oral lesions of epidermolysis bullosa acquisita.

Suggested Therapies

Systemic Treatment

Oral Corticosteroids

Oral corticosteroids (prednisone or prednisolone) 30–100 mg/day, depending on the disease severity, may temporarily control the disease. Once clinical control is achieved, the dose is gradually tapered to 5–10 mg/day. Recurrences are common.

Immunosuppressive Agents

Immunosuppressive agents such as azathioprine 50–150 mg/day, cyclophosphamide 100–200 mg/day, cyclosporine 5–9 mg/kg per day, mycophenolate mofetil 2 g/day, either alone or more commonly as adjuvant therapy to the oral corticosteroids may be used, but their benefit is uncertain. In addition, the significant side effects of immunosuppressive agents must always be taken into account.

Colchicine

Colchicine 0.5–2 mg/day for 4–6 months has been used successfully in patients with limited or mild disease or refractory epidermolysis bullosa acquisita. The drug may be used alone or in combination with oral corticosteroids.

Intravenous Immunoglobulin

Recently, high-doses i.v. immunoglobulin 400 mg/kg per day given over 5 days at 4–6-week intervals has been suggested as the best choice for severe, resistant disease, especially with mucosal involvement.

Topical Treatment

Localized oral lesions may be controlled with application of topical corticosteroids in adhesive paste (triamcinolone acetonide, fluocinolone acetonide, clobetasol propionate). Oral paste with 0.1 % tacrolimus may also be effective. High-potency topical corticosteroids may be used for localized skin lesions. Nonspecific supportive measures should be employed to control cutaneous infection.

Alternative Therapies

These include dapsone, plasmapheresis, and extracorporeal photochemotherapy.

References

Camara A, Becherel PA, Bussel A, et al. Resistant acquired bullous epidermolysis with severe ocular involvement: the success of extracorporal photochemotherapy. *Ann Dermatol Venereol* 1999;126:612–615.

Cunningham BB, Kirchmann TT, Woodley D. Colchicine for epidermolysis bullosa acquisita. *J Am Acad Dermatol* 1996;34:781–784.

Engineer L, Ahmed AR. Emerging treatment for epidermolysis bullosa acquisita. *J Am Acad Dermatol* 2001;44: 818–828.

Hallel-Halevy D, Nadelman C, Chen M, Woodley DT. Epidermolysis bullosa acquisita: Update and review. *Clin Dermatol* 2001;19:712–718.

Harman KE, Whittam LR, Wakeling SH, Black MM. Severe, refractory epidermolysis bullosa complicated by an oesophageal stricture responding to intravenous immune globulin. *Br J Dermatol* 1998;139:1126–1127.

Hughes AP, Callen JP. Epidermolysis bullosa acquisita responsive to dapsone therapy. *J Cutan Med Surg* 2001;5:397–399.

Jolles S. High-dose intravenous immunoglobulin (hdIVIg) in the treatment of autoimmune blistering disorders. *Clin Exp Immunol* 2002;129:385–389.

Khatri ML, Benhazeil M, Shafi M. Epidermolysis bullosa acquisita responsive to cyclosporin therapy. *J Eur Acad Dermatol Venereol* 2000;15:182–184.

Kofler H, Wambacher-Gasser B, Topar G, et al. Intravenous immunoglobulin treatment in therapy-resistant epidermolysis bullosa acquisita. *J Am Acad Dermatol* 1996;34:331–335.

Korman NJ. New immunomodulating drugs in autoimmune blistering diseases. *Dermatol Clin* 2001;19:637–648.

Trebing D, Ziemer A. Acquired epidermolysis bullosa with a highly varied clinical picture and successful treatment with mycophenolate mofetil. *Hautarzt* 2001;52:717–721.

Epulis Fissuratum

Definition

Epulis fissuratum is a relatively common hyperplastic, fibrous connective tissue lesion.

Etiology

Epulis fissuratum is caused by ill-fitting dentures or dentures that are worn for long periods of time.

Main Clinical Features

- Hyperplastic tissue clinically present as multiple tissue folds usually in the anterior alveolar vestibule. The tissues of the lesion are of normal color and are firm in texture
- Painful ulceration is common at the base of the fold

Diagnosis

The diagnosis is based on the clinical features. Biopsy and histopathologic examination is occasionally necessary to rule out malignancy.

Differential Diagnosis

- Squamous cell carcinoma
- Multiple fibromas
- Pyogenic granuloma
- Neurofibromatosis

Treatment

- Surgical excision of the hyperplastic tissue as well as denture adjustment or fabrication of a new denture is recommended.
- CO_2 laser surgery may also be used.

References

Buchner A, Begleiter A, Hansen LS. The predominance of epulis fissuratum in females. *Quintessence Int* 1984;15:699–702.

Coelho CM, Zucoloto S, Lopez RA. Denture-induced fibrous inflammatory hyperplasia: A retrospective study in a school of dentistry. *Int J Prosthodont* 2000;13:148–151.

Cutright DE. The histopathologic findings in 583 cases of epulis fissuratum. *Oral Surg Oral Med Oral Pathol* 1974;37:401–411.

Keng SB, Loh HS. The treatment of epulis fissuratum of the oral cavity by CO_2 laser surgery. *J Clin Laser Med Surg* 1992;10:303–306.

Meister F Jr, Hickman TR, Davies EE. Surgical treatment of epulis fissuratum utilizing free gingival grafts: Report of two cases. *J Wiscon Dent Assoc* 1977;53:257–259.

Scholle RH, Tiecke RW. Perspectives in patient care: Epulis fissuratum. *Illinois Dent J* 1975;44:28–30.

Erythema Multiforme

▨ Definition

Erythema multiforme is an acute, self-limiting, mucocutaneous disease that more frequently affects young individuals and, less often, adults and the elderly.

▨ Etiology

A number of etiologic factors have been implicated including herpes simplex virus, *Mycoplasma pneumoniae*, and drugs. Erythema multiforme is currently considered an immunologic disease.

▨ Main Clinical Features

There are two main clinical variants: a) erythema multiforme minor and b) erythema multiforme major or Stevens–Johnson syndrome. The disease recurs in 20–30% of the cases.

Minor Erythema Multiforme

Oral Mucosa

It is involved in about 20–30% of cases. Rarely, it may be the only manifestation. The lesions appear as multiple small vesicles that rupture, leaving extensive painful erosions covered by whitish pseudomembranes

Other Mucosae

Rarely conjunctiva, genital mucosa

Skin

The skin lesions are almost always present as erythematous maculopapules, usually presenting as numerous characteristic *target or iris-like* lesions. Less often pruritic plaques and bullae may appear. The duration of the lesions varies from 1 to 4 weeks

Major Erythema Multiforme

Oral Mucosa

The oral mucosa lesions are severe and almost always present. The initial lesions appear as erythematous areas, evolving soon into vesicles that rapidly rupture leaving painful erosions covered by yellowish-white pseudomembranes or hemorrhagic crusts

Other Mucosae

Ocular, genital, pharynx, larynx, esophagus, and bronchial mucosae are usually involved with severe lesions

Skin

Cutaneous involvement is contemporaneous or, more frequently, subsequent to that of the mucosae and may be seen as figurate erythematous–edematous lesions, with blisters evolving to erosions with massive denudation of the epidermis or with target lesions. The skin lesions are usually characterized by lack of symmetry, involvement of nontypical areas and longer duration

▨ Diagnosis

The diagnosis of erythema multiforme is based on clinical and histopathologic criteria.

▨ Differential Diagnosis

- Primary herpetic gingivostomatitis
- Herpetiform ulcers
- Bullous pemphigoid
- Cicatricial pemphigoid
- Linear IgA disease
- Pemphigoid gestationis
- Pemphigus
- Epidermolysis bullosa acquisita
- Other drug eruptions

▨ Treatment

Basic Guidelines

- The management should include identification and elimination of any possible inciting infection or drug.

- Most cases of minor erythema multiforme are self-limiting and need only symptomatic treatment.
- The use of systemic corticosteroids is currently controversial. However, we believe that corticosteroids in low doses are helpful, particularly for the oral lesions.
- In major erythema multiforme bed rest or hospital management is recommended.
- Antiviral therapy may eliminate recurrence in some cases.

Suggested Therapies

Systemic Treatment

Oral Corticosteroids

Early use of corticosteroids, during the first 2–4 days, usually reduces the period of acute eruption and symptoms. For minor erythema multiforme 20–40 mg/day prednisone or prednisolone administered for 4–6 days usually control the disease. The dose is then quickly tapered and completely stopped not later than 2 weeks. Major erythema multiforme usually requires doses of 40–80 mg/day with gradual tapering over 2–3 weeks.

Antibiotics

Antibiotics (e.g., erythromycin 0.5–1 g three times per day) are necessary if a secondary infection is present or if there are indications that the disease is associated with *Mycoplasma pneumoniae*.

Antiviral Agents

Oral acyclovir 400 mg twice a day for 4–6 months is indicated in some recurrent cases, when herpes simplex virus is suspected to be responsible. Newer antiviral agents (valacyclovir 500 mg/day for 4–6 months, or famciclovir 250 mg twice daily for 4–6 months) may also be effective.

Topical Treatment

Careful oral hygiene, soft diet, topical anesthetic agents (lidocaine [Xylocaine] gel, benzocaine lozenges), antiseptic mouthwash with hydrogen peroxide or chlorhexidine, topical corticosteroids, e. g., 0.1 % triamcinolone acetonide paste or 0.05 % clobetasol propionate ointment may help to eliminate discomfort.

Alternative Therapies

Levamisole 100–150 mg/day, thalidomide 100–200 mg/day, azathioprine 100 mg/day, cyclophosphamide 100–150 mg/day, and dapsone 50–100 mg/day have been used mainly in chronic and recurrent disease.

References

Esterly NB. Corticosteroids for erythema multiforme? *Pediatr Dermatol* 1989;6:229–250.

Fabbri P, Panconesi E. Erythema multiforme "minus" and "mains" and drug intake. *Clin Dermatol* 1993;11:479–489.

Farthing PM, Maragaou P, Coates M, et al. Characteristics of the oral lesions in patients with cutaneous recurrent erythema multiforme. *J Oral Pathol Med* 1995;24:9–13.

Lozada-Nur F, Corsky M, Silverman S Jr. Oral erythema multiforme: Clinical observations and treatment of 95 patients. *Oral Surg Oral Med Oral Pathol* 1989;67:36–40.

Moisson YF, Janier M, Civatte J. Thalidomide for recurrent erythema multiforme. *Br J Dermatol* 1992;126:92–93.

Patterson R, Miller M, Kaplan M, et al. Stevens–Johnson syndrome: Effectiveness of corticosteroids in management and recurrent Stevens–Johnson syndrome. *Allergy Proc* 1992;13:89–95.

Rasmussen JE. Erythema multiforme: Should anyone care about the standards of care? *Arch Dermatol* 1995;131:726–729.

Tatnall FM, Schofield JK, Leigh IM. A double blind, placebo controlled trial of continuous acyclovir therapy in recurrent erythema multiforme. *Br J Dermatol* 1995;132:267–270.

Erythroplakia

Definition

Erythroplakia or erythroplasia of Queyrat is a rare and dangerous precancerous lesion, characterized by a red nonspecific plaque on the oral mucosa that cannot be attributed to any other known disease.

Etiology

The etiology of erythroplakia is unknown. Predisposing factors are mainly smoking, alcohol, and human papillomavirus (HPV).

Main Clinical Features

Erythroplakia mainly involves the glans penis. Oral involvement is rare.

- Fiery red, slightly elevated or flat plaque of varying size
- Occasionally multiple white spots may be present in or peripheral to the erythematous area
- Smooth and velvety surface
- Usually asymptomatic
- More than 90–95 % of cases of erythroplakia demonstrate histologically severe epithelial dysplasia, carcinoma in situ or invasive squamous cell carcinoma at the times of diagnosis

Diagnosis

Biopsy and histopathologic examination confirms the diagnosis and determines the risk for carcinoma.

Differential Diagnosis

- Speckled leukoplakia
- Erythematous candidiasis
- Early squamous cell carcinoma
- Mucositis
- Local irritation
- Lichen planus
- Lupus erythematosus
- Median rhomboid glossitis
- Drug reactions

Treatment

Basic Guidelines

- Biopsy and histopathologic examination must be done before treatment.
- Elimination of predisposing factors thought to be involved in the pathogenesis.
- Improvement of oral hygiene.
- Long-term follow-up of the patients is important after treatment as recurrences are common.

Suggested Therapies

- Surgical management is the mainstay of treatment of erythroplakia. The extent of excision depends on the histopathologic findings.
- Interventional laser surgery is an alternative treatment for oral erythroplakia.
- Radiation and chemotherapy may be used as adjunctive and palliative treatments in advanced cases with squamous cell carcinoma.
- Topical 5 % imiquimod cream and 5-aminolevulinic acid photodynamic therapy have been used with success in the treatment of erythroplakia of the glans penis.

References

Kaspari M, Gutzmer R, Kiehl P, et al. Imiquimod 5 % cream in the treatment of human papillomavirus-16-positive erythroplasia of Queyrat. *Dermatology* 2002;205:67–69.

Porter WM, Francis N, Hawkins D, et al. Penile intraepithelial neoplasia: Clinical spectrum and treatment of 35 cases. *Br J Dermatol* 2002;147:1159–1165.

Sciubba JJ. Oral cancer. The importance of early diagnosis and treatment. *Am J Clin Dermatol* 2001;2:239–251.

Stables GI, Stringer MR, Robinson DJ, Ash DV. Erythroplasia of Queyrat treated by topical aminolaevulinic acid photodynamic therapy. *Br J Dermatol* 1999;142:825–826.

Thomson PJ, Wylie J. Interventional laser surgery: an effective surgical and diagnostic tool in oral precancer management. *Int J Oral Maxillofac Surg* 2002;31:145–153.

Exfoliative Cheilitis

◾ Definition

Exfoliative cheilitis is a chronic inflammatory disorder of the vermilion border of the lips.

◾ Etiology

The etiology is unknown. The disorder is most commonly observed in young females with emotional stress and a history of atopic dermatitis. It is also relatively common in HIV-infected patients. Cold and hot weather usually worsen the condition.

◾ Main Clinical Features

- Exfoliation of the vermilion border of the lips, leaving an erythematous and sensitive surface
- Chronic dryness, scaling and cracking of the vermilion border of the lips
- The lesions may persist with varying severity for months or years, with remissions and exacerbations
- Severe cases may cause cosmetic problems for the patients

◾ Diagnosis

The diagnosis is based on the history and the clinical features.

◾ Differential Diagnosis

- Cheilitis due to retinoids
- Contact cheilitis
- Actinic cheilitis
- Plasma cell cheilitis
- Infectious cheilitis
- Psoriasis of the lips

◾ Treatment

Basic Guidelines

- Elimination of emotional stress.
- Patients should be advised to avoid self-irritation, lip sucking and licking, and exposure to the wind and cold and very hot weather.

Suggested Therapies

- Topical moistening agents and low-potency corticosteroid ointments usually improve the condition. However, recurrences are common.
- Systemic oral corticosteroids in low doses, e. g., prednisone 10–15 mg/day for about 2–3 weeks and then tapering the dose to 5 mg/day for 2–4 weeks usually controls the disease activity.
- Topical immunomodulators, such as tacrolimus and 0.1 % pimecrolimus ointment in my experience were seen to be effective in a group of patients with exfoliative cheilitis. Their use is safe with minor local side effects such as burning, itching, and erythema.

References

Casariego Z, Pombo T, Perez H, Patterson P. Eruptive cheilitis: A new adverse effect in reactive HIV-positive patients subjected to high activity antiretroviral therapy (HAART): presentation of six clinical cases. *Med Oral* 2001;6:19–30.

Daley TD, Gupta AK. Exfoliative cheilitis. *J Oral Pathol Med* 1995;24:177–179.

Laskaris G. *Color Atlas of Oral Diseases*, 3rd edition. Thieme Verlag: Stuttgart, 2003.

Ramirez-Amador V, Esquirel-Pedraza L, Mohar A, et al. Chemotherapy-associated oral mucosal lesions in patients with leukemia or lymphoma. *Eur J Cancer B Oral Oncol* 1996;32B:322–327.

Reichart PA, Weigel D, Schmidt-Westhausen A, Pohle HD. Exfoliative cheilitis in AIDS: association with *Candida* infection. *J Oral Pathol Med* 1997;26:290–293.

Extramedullary Oral Plasmacytoma

▓ Definition

Extramedullary oral soft tissue plasmacytoma is an unusual neoplasm of plasma cell origin.

▓ Etiology

The etiology of extramedullary oral plasmacytoma is unknown.

▓ Main Clinical Features

- Lesion presents as painless nonspecific soft tissue swelling
- Surface of the lesion is smooth with normal color, but it may ultimately ulcerate
- Size varies from 1 cm to several centimeters in diameter
- Oral mucosa is rarely affected; the gingiva and the palate are more frequently involved

▓ Diagnosis

The clinical diagnosis should be confirmed by a biopsy and histopathologic examination and immunohistochemical evaluation.

▓ Differential Diagnosis

- Non-Hodgkin lymphomas
- Multiple myeloma
- Necrotizing sialadenometaplasia
- Pyogenic granuloma
- Pleomorphic adenoma
- Other benign salivary gland tumors
- Malignant salivary gland neoplasms

▓ Treatment

- Surgical excision is the treatment of choice for solitary localized lesions.
- Radiotherapy at a dose of 4000–5000 cGy is also effective. Combined radiation therapy and chemotherapy may also be used in more severe cases.
- Thalidomide in combination with cyclophosphamide and dexamethasone is effective in soft-tissue plasmacytoma.

References

Blade J, Esteve J, Rosinol L, et al. Thalidomide in refractory and relapsing multiple myeloma. *Semin Oncol* 2001;28: 588–592.

Dimopoulos MA, Kiamuris C, Moulopoulos LA. Solitary plasmacytoma of bone and extramedullary plasmacytoma. *Hematol Oncol Clin North Am* 1999;13:1249–1257.

Gonzalez-Porras JR, Gonzalez M, et al. Thalidomide in combination with cyclophosphamide and dexamethasone (Tracydex) is effective in soft-tissue plasmacytoma. *Br J Haematol* 2002;119:883–884.

Mendenhall WM, Mendenhall CM, Mendenhall NP. Solitary plasmacytoma of bone and soft tissues. *Am J Otolaryngol* 2003;24:395–399.

Michalaki VJ, Hall J, Henk JM, et al. Definitive radiotherapy for extramedullary plasmacytomas of the head and neck. *Br J Radiol* 2000;76:738–741.

Tsang RW, Gospodarowicz MK, Pintilie M, et al. Solitary plasmacytoma treated with radiotherapy: Impact of tumor size on outcome. *Int J Radiat Oncol Biol Phys* 2001;50:113–120.

FAPA Syndrome

Definition

FAPA syndrome is a rare oral disease characterized by periodic fever, aphthous ulcers, pharyngitis, and cervical adenitis.

Etiology

The etiology is unknown. However, an immune mechanism may be involved in the pathogenesis.

Main Clinical Features

- High fever (39–40 °C) lasting 4–6 days associated by chills and malaise
- Aphthous ulcers, minor or major type
- Pharyngitis and tonsillitis
- Bilateral cervical lymphadenopathy
- Headache, abdominal pain, and arthralgia may be present
- Disease usually recurs at fixed intervals of every 4–8 weeks
- Children below 10 years are more frequently affected

Diagnosis

The diagnosis is based on the medical history and the clinical features.

Differential Diagnosis

- Aphthous ulcers
- Behçet disease
- Primary herpetic gingivostomatitis
- Sweet syndrome
- Cyclic neutropenia
- Leukemia
- HIV infection

Treatment

Basic Guidelines

- Children should stay in bed for 4–5 days.
- Soft foods and drinks are necessary during the acute phase.
- Antipyretics should be given during the high-fever period.
- There is no absolutely successful treatment.

Suggested Therapies

- Cimetidine, as an immunomodulating agent in a dose of 20–30 mg/kg per day for about a week usually helps to improve the signs and symptoms of the syndrome.
- Oral corticosteroids in low doses, e.g., prednisone 10–20 mg/day for 3–6 days may also be used as a second-line choice.
- Nonsteroidal anti-inflammatory agents have also been used.

References

Feder HM Jr. Periodic fever, aphthous stomatiits, pharyngitis, adenitis: A clinical review of a new syndrome. *Curr Opin Pediatr* 2000;12:253–256.

Kawashima H, Nishimata S, Shimizu T, et al. Highly suspected case of FAPA syndrome. *Pediatr Int* 2001;43: 103–106.

Padeh S, Brezniak N, Zemer D, et al. Periodic fever, aphthous stomatitis, pharyngitis, and adenopathy syndrome: Clinical characteristic and outcome. *J Pediatr* 1999;135:98–101.

Pillet P, Ansoborio S, Carrere A, et al. FAPA syndrome: Interet de la cimetidine. *Arch Pediatr* 2000;7:54–57.

Fissured Tongue

Definition

Fissured or scrotal tongue is a common benign condition of the dorsum of the tongue.

Etiology

The etiology is unknown. However, heredity appears to play a significant role.

Main Clinical Features

- Multiple fissures or grooves on the dorsum of the tongue
- The grooves vary in depth, size, and number
- Usually asymptomatic
- Usually coexists with geographic tongue and may be a component of Melkersson–Rosenthal syndrome, Down syndrome, and Sjögren syndrome

Diagnosis

The diagnosis is exclusively based on the clinical features.

Differential Diagnosis

- Sjögren syndrome
- Melkersson–Rosenthal syndrome
- Interstitial syphilitic glossitis

Treatment

- Fissured tongue is a benign condition requiring no treatment. Patients should be reassured.
- Brushing the dorsum of the tongue with a soft toothbrush (tongue cleaner) may be occasionally suggested because food debris can be entrapped in the fissures and produce slight irritation.

References

Laskaris G. *Color Atlas of Oral Diseases*, 3rd edition. Thieme Verlag: Stuttgart, 2003.

Focal Epithelial Hyperplasia

■ Definition

Focal epithelial hyperplasia or Heck disease is a benign, hyperplastic viral disease of the oral mucosa.

■ Etiology

The causative organisms are human papillomavirus types 13 and 32.

■ Main Clinical Features

The disease involves the oral mucosa and is more common in children, exhibiting a racial predilection (Eskimos, North American Indians, South Africans, and rarely Europeans and Asians).

- Multiple painless, sessile, slightly elevated, soft nodules 1–10 mm in diameter
- Lesion surface is smooth with a whitish or normal color
- Characteristically, on stretching the mucosa the lesions tend to disappear
- Lips, buccal mucosa, tongue, and gingiva are more frequently affected

■ Diagnosis

Histopathologic examination confirms the diagnosis. In-situ hybridization may also be helpful.

■ Differential Diagnosis

- Condylomata acuminata
- Verruca vulgaris
- Multiple papillomas
- Multiple fibromas
- Focal dermal hypoplasia syndrome
- Oral lesions of Cowden disease
- Oral lesions of tuberous sclerosis

■ Treatment

Basic Guidelines

- The lesions may occasionally regress spontaneously without treatment.
- There is no specific antiviral therapy.

Suggested Therapies

- Invasive therapies such as electrosurgery, surgical excision, cryotherapy, and CO_2 laser are the therapies of choice for focal epithelial hyperplasia depending on the number of lesions and the sites affected.
- Systemic interferon alpha-2a and -2b alone or in combination with CO_2 laser have been used with success in multifocal lesions.
- Recently, successful treatment of focal epithelial hyperplasia with topical interferon beta (Fiblaferon gel) applied five times daily for about 12 weeks have been reported. This alternative therapeutic regimen is simple and noninvasive, but trials with large series of patients with the disease are required to confirm that it is effective.

References

Akyol A, Anadolu R, Anadoly Y, et al. Multifocal papillomavirus epithelial hyperplasia: Successful treatment with CO_2 laser therapy combined with interferon alpha-2b. *Int J Dermatol* 2003;42:733–735.

Bassioukas K, Danielides V, Georgiou I, et al. Oral focal epithelial hyperplasia. *Eur J Dermatol* 2000;10:395–397.

Kose O, Akar A, Safali M, et al. Focal epithelial hyperplasia treated with interferon alpha-2a. *J Dermatol Treat* 2001;12:111–113.

Laskaris G, Papanicolaou S, et al. Focal epithelial hyperplasia: The first reported case from Greece. *Dermatologica* 1981;162:254–258.

Steinhoff M, Metze D, Stockfleth E, Luger TA. Successful topical treatment of focal epithelial hyperplasia (Heck's disease) with interferon-β. *Br J Dermatol* 2001;144: 1067–1069.

Furred Tongue

Definition

Furred or coated tongue is a common benign disorder of the tongue particularly in individuals with painful oral lesions or febrile illnesses.

Etiology

The predisposing factors are poor oral hygiene, soft diet, and dehydration. The coating is a mixture of lengthened and keratotic filiform papillae, food debris, and microbial elements.

Main Clinical Features

- White or whitish-yellow thick coating on the dorsum of the tongue
- Unpleasant taste and xerostomia are common symptoms
- Characteristically, furred tongue appears and disappears quickly

Diagnosis

The diagnosis is exclusively based on the medical history and clinical features.

Differential Diagnosis

- Hairy tongue
- Candidiasis
- Hairy leukoplakia
- Chemical burns

Treatment

- Treatment of the underlying illnesses.
- Hydration.
- Good oral hygiene.
- Mechanical scraping of the dorsum of the tongue by a tongue cleaner.

References

Darwazeh AM, Pillai K. Prevalence of tongue lesions in 1013 Jordanian dental outpatients. *Comm Dent Oral Epidemiol* 1993;21:323–324.

Laskaris G. *Color Atlas of Oral Diseases*, 3rd edition. Thieme Verlag: Stuttgart, 2003.

Geographic Tongue

Definition

Geographic tongue or benign migratory glossitis is a common benign inflammatory disorder of the tongue. Rarely, similar lesions may develop on the lip or buccal mucosa and palate.

Etiology

The etiology is unknown, although an inherited pattern is possible.

Main Clinical Features

- Demarcated red areas of the dorsal and lateral tongue with scalloped thin white borders
- Lesions are usually multiple although a solitary lesion may occur
- Characteristically the lesions persist for a short time in one area then disappear and reappear later on another area of the tongue
- Geographic tongue is usually asymptomatic. However, some patients may occasionally complain of a burning sensation and sensitivity to hot and spicy foods

Diagnosis

The diagnosis is exclusively based on the clinical features.

Differential Diagnosis

- Oral psoriasis
- Reiter syndrome
- Candidiasis
- Leukoplakia
- Lichen planus
- Cinnamon contact glossitis
- Mucous patches of syphilis
- Plasma cell glossitis

Treatment

- Geographic tongue usually requires no treatment. The patients should be assured that the disorder is benign.
- If subjective symptoms are present, avoidance of hot and spicy foods and increased intake of foods rich in ascorbic acid is advisable. The use of chamomile mouthwashes several times daily for 2–3 weeks usually provides relief of the symptoms.
- In more severe and persistent cases low- or medium-potency topical corticosteroid gels may be helpful.

References

Fenerli A, Papanikolaou S, Papanikolaou M, Laskaris G. Histocompatibility antigens and geographic tongue. *Oral Surg Oral Med Oral Pathol* 1995;76:476–479.

Laskaris G. *Color Atlas of Oral Diseases*, 3rd edition. Thieme Verlag: Stuttgart, 2003.

Glossodynia

Definition

Glossodynia or glossopyrosis or burning mouth syndrome is one of the most common oral problems. It is not a specific disease entity but a symptom of burning sensation of the tongue with no clinically visible changes.

Etiology

In the great majority of the cases glossodynia represents a symptom of an underlying psychological problem. Other causes are iron deficiency anemia, pernicious anemia, lichen planus, xerostomia, diabetes mellitus, candidiasis, and a host of other diseases.

Main Clinical Features

- No clinically visible changes
- Burning sensation or itching, usually at the tip and the lateral borders of the tongue
- Similar symptoms may appear in other oral sites
- Dry mouth and bad taste may occur
- Symptoms show remissions and exacerbations and may persist for months or years
- Patients usually develop cancerophobia

Diagnosis

The diagnosis is exclusively based on the medical history and the clinical features.

Differential Diagnosis

- Iron-deficiency anemia
- Plummer–Vinson syndrome
- Pernicious anemia
- Lichen planus
- Diabetes mellitus
- Candidiasis
- Sjögren syndrome

- Contact stomatitis
- Neurologic disorders
- Collagen diseases
- Drug-induced side effects
- Vitamin deficiencies

Treatment

Basic Guidelines

- Any visible or systemic disease which can produce glossodynia should be ruled out.
- Help the patients to rid themselves of cancerophobia or AIDS-phobia and to understand that psychological factors are responsible for the symptom.
- Collaboration with the patient's psychiatrist is mandatory.

Suggested Therapies

- Chamomile mouthwash four to five times daily over a long period of time may improves the symptom.
- Avoid any pharmaceutical mouthwash products as they usually worsen the problem.
- Mild tranquilizers and antidepressants may be helpful in more severe cases although such agents must be prescribed by a psychiatrist.

References

Bessho K, Okubo Y, Hori S, et al. Effectiveness of kampo medicine (sai-boku-to) in treatment of patients with glossodynia. *Oral Surg Oral Med Oral Pathol Oral Radiol Endod* 1998;86:678–681.

Gorsky M, Silverman S, Chinn H. Clinical characteristics and management outcome in burning mouth syndrome. *Oral Surg Oral Med Oral Pathol* 1991;72:192–195.

Maresky LS, van der Bijl P, Gird I. Burning mouth syndrome. Evaluation of multiple variables among 85 patients. *Oral Surg Oral Med Oral Pathol* 1993;75:303–307.

Meiss F, Boerner D, Marsch WC, Fischer M. Gabapentin: A promising treatment of glossodynia. *Clin Exp Dermatol* 2002;27:525–526.

Tanaka M, Kitago H, Ogawa S, et al. Incidence and treatment of dysgeusia in patients with glossodynia. *Acta Otolaryngol Suppl* 2002;546:142–145.

Gonococcal Stomatitis

▨ Definition

Gonorrhea or gonococcal infection is a common sexually transmitted disease that primarily involves mucous membranes and leads to urethritis, cervicitis, proctitis, and oropharyngitis.

▨ Etiology

The causative organism is the Gram-negative diplococcus *Neisseria gonorrhoeae.*

▨ Main Clinical Features

Gonococcal stomatitis and pharyngitis are rare and the result of oral sex.

Oral Lesions

- Nonspecific clinical signs and symptoms
- Redness and inflammation
- Rarely erosions and ulcers covered with a whitish pseudomembrane
- Itching and burning in the involved areas
- Oral gonococcal infection may be asymptomatic

Pharyngeal Lesions

- Sore throat
- Diffuse or patchy erythema and edema
- Tiny pustules on the tonsillar pillars and uvula

▨ Diagnosis

Gram stain and culture are always necessary for final diagnosis. Serologic tests are of limited use.

▨ Differential Diagnosis

- Streptococcal stomatitis
- Herpetic stomatitis
- Candidiasis
- Lichen planus
- Cinnamon contact stomatitis
- Thermal and chemical burns

▨ Treatment

Basic Guidelines

- Only those patients with oral lesions and positive microscopy and culture or those who have had recent oral sex with a partner with confirmed gonorrhea should be treated.
- Oral gonococcal stomatitis should be treated with systemic antibiotics.
- Oropharyngeal gonococcal infection frequently resolves spontaneously within a few weeks.
- The choice of antibiotics depends on the resistance of the microorganism, the anatomic area infected, side effects of the drugs and the cost.
- During the past two decades resistance of *N. gonorrhoeae* to penicillin, erythromycin, and tetracyclines has continued to exist.

Suggested Therapies

A single-dose regimen of oral ciprofloxacin 500 mg, or ofloxacin 400 mg, or cefixime 400 mg is recommended for oral and pharyngeal gonococcal infection. This therapeutic regimen has good efficacy and safety.

Alternative Therapies

All these regimens are recommended for patients with gonococcal infection of the urethra, cervix, and rectum and not for oropharyngeal infection. Penicillin, amoxicillin, or spectinomycin may be used as the alternative treatment.

References

Fitzgerald M, Bedford C. National standards for the management of gonorrhoea. *Int J STD AIDS* 1996;7:298–300.

Hutt DM, Judson FN. Epidemiology and treatment of oropharyngeal gonorrhoea. *Ann Intern Med* 1986;104: 655–658.

Moran JS, Levine WC. Drugs of choice for the treatment of uncomplicated gonococcal infections. *Clin Infect Dis* 1995;20:547–565.

Moran JS. Treating uncomplicated *Neisseria gonorrhoeae* infections: Is the anatomic site of infection important? *Sex Transm Dis* 1995;22:39–47.

Graft-Versus-Host Disease

▧ Definition

Graft-versus-host disease (GVHD) is one of the major complications of allogeneic bone marrow or peripheral blood stem cell transplantation.

▧ Etiology

It is a complex multisystemic disorder in which specific immunologic phenomena may occur as well as nonspecific features may be present.

▧ Classification

Graft-versus-host disease is classically divided into two types:
- Acute, which occurs between 1 and 3 weeks after transplantation, but it may develop by 3 months and occurs in 25–50% of patients.
- Chronic, which develops usually after 3 months posttransplantation and occurs in 40–50% of patients.

▧ Main Clinical Features

Oral lesions may develop either in the acute or chronic form and the prevalence varies from 50% to 80%. Oral lesions are more common in the chronic form of the disease. In some patients the oral lesions may be the only manifestation.

Oral Lesions

Acute Form
- Diffuse erythema and painful ulcerations of the oral mucosa
- Hemorrhage, xerostomia
- Lichenoid lesions
- Viral, bacterial, and fungal infections

Chronic Form
- Diffuse lichenoid lesions
- Multiple painful ulcerations
- Superficial mucocoeles, pyogenic granuloma, and verruciform xanthomas may be present
- Xerostomia and Sjögren-like syndrome
- Fibrosis and limitation of mouth opening

- Viral, bacterial, and fungal infections are common

Other Manifestations

Acute Form
- High fever
- Hepatic failure and gastrointestinal symptoms
- Generalized, erythematous, maculopapular rash
- Rarely bullae formation and skin desquamation develop
- Infections

Chronic Form
- Liver, pulmonary, gastrointestinal, and conjunctival disorders
- Musculoskeletal disorders
- Lichenoid skin lesions
- Scleroderma-like skin lesions
- Skin hypermelanosis
- Severe infections

▧ Diagnosis

The diagnosis is mainly based on the medical history and clinical features. Biopsy and histopathologic examination of labial salivary glands and oral mucosa are helpful.

▧ Differential Diagnosis

- Drug-induced stomatitis
- Lichen planus
- Lupus erythematosus
- Scleroderma
- Erythema multiforme
- Sjögren syndrome
- Pemphigus
- Pemphigoid
- Neutropenia-associated mucositis
- Radiation mucositis

▒ Treatment

Basic Guidelines

- All patients should have oral and dental evaluation before transplantation.
- Eliminate active oral and dental infections and any source of trauma (mobile teeth, broken teeth, and restorations).
- Establish an appropriate level of oral hygiene for the patient.
- Mouthwashes containing alcohol and flavoring agents should be avoided as they increase the symptoms.
- Gentle brushing of the dorsum of the tongue with a soft tongue cleaner.
- There should be close cooperation between the oral clinician and the transplantation specialist before any treatment of oral lesions of graft-versus-host disease is commenced.
- The main role in the treatment of graft-versus-host disease is of the specialist.

Suggested Therapies

- Topical rinses with 0.9% saline solution and sodium bicarbonate solution may be used several times daily. Hydrogen peroxide rinses may also be used.
- Topical anesthetics, e.g., 2% lidocaine or benzocaine are of limited help.
- Topical corticosteroids (ointments, elixirs, gels) are helpful in cases with oral ulcerations.

- Artificial saliva and systemic sialogogues may be used in patients with xerostomia.
- Systemic oral corticosteroids (increase the dose in patients already on them) are recommended in patients with severe oral ulceration and the chronic form of graft-versus-host disease. This treatment should be undertaken in collaboration with the specialist.
- Prevention or treatment of oral infections (viral, bacterial, and fungal) is indicated with the appropriate therapeutic regimen.
- Cyclosporine, tacrolimus, methotrexate, azathioprine, mycophenolate mofetil, and corticosteroids are the drugs used in various prophylactic regimens in patients undergoing bone marrow or stem cell transplantation.

References

Barker GJ. Current practices in the oral management of the patient undergoing chemotherapy or bone marrow transplantation. *Support Care Cancer* 1999;7:17–20.

Majorana A, Schubert MM, Porta F, et al. Oral complications of pediatric hematopoietic cell transplantation: Diagnosis and management. *Support Care Cancer* 2000;8:353–365.

Schubert MM, Sullivan KM. Recognition, incidence, and management of oral graft-versus-host disease. *Natl Cancer Inst Monogr* 1990;9:135–144.

Woo S-B, Sonis ST, Monopoli MM, Sonis AL. A longitudinal study of oral ulcerative mucositis in bone marrow transplant recipients. *Cancer* 1993;72:1612–1617.

Hairy Leukoplakia

Definition

Hairy leukoplakia is a unique oral mucosal lesion which occurs in HIV-infected patients and rarely in immunocompromised individuals.

Etiology

The Epstein–Barr virus has been implicated in the etiology.

Main Clinical Features

- Whitish, slightly elevated, nonremovable lesions
- Surface of the lesion is corrugated with a vertical orientation
- Lesions are painless and asymptomatic
- Lesions usually appear bilaterally on the lateral borders of the tongue and rarely in other areas of the oral cavity

Diagnosis

The diagnosis should be confirmed by biopsy and histopathologic examination and polymerase chain reaction (PCR).

Differential Diagnosis

- Candidiasis
- Leukoedema
- Chronic biting
- Cinnamon contact stomatitis
- Leukoplakia
- Lichen planus
- Lupus erythematosus
- Uremic stomatitis
- Geographic tongue
- Oral psoriasis
- White sponge nevus

Treatment

Basic Guidelines

- Hairy leukoplakia is an asymptomatic benign lesion.
- Treatment is usually not necessary except for psychologic and aesthetic reasons.
- Topical use of keratolytic agents should be avoided.
- The lesions tend to recur when treatment is discontinued.

Suggested Therapies

- Oral acyclovir 400–800 mg four times daily for about 1 month or more is the drug of choice and is usually effective.
- Valacyclovir 500–1000 mg twice daily for 1–2 months or famciclovir 250 mg three times daily for 1 month or more may also be used with success.
- Hairy leukoplakia usually regresses during highly active antiretroviral therapy (HAART).

References

Greenspan D, Shirlaw PJ. Management of the oral mucosal lesions seen in association with HIV infection. *Oral Dis* 1997;3(suppl 1):S229–S234.

Laskaris G. Oral manifestation of HIV disease. *Clin Dermatol* 2000;18:447–455.

Laskaris G, Laskaris M, Theodoridou M. Oral hairy leukoplakia in a child with AIDS. *Oral Surg Oral Med Oral Pathol* 1995;79:570–571.

Reichart PA. Clinical management of selected oral fungal and viral infections during HIV-disease. *Int Dent J* 1999;49:251–259.

Walling DM, Flaitz CM, Nichols CM. Epstein–Barr virus replication in oral hairy leukoplakia: Response, persistence, and resistance to treatment with valacyclovir. *J Infect Dis* 2003;188:883–890.

Hairy Tongue

Definition

Hairy tongue is a common benign disorder of the dorsum of the tongue due to keratin accumulation, hypertrophy, and elongation of the filiform papillae.

Etiology

The etiology is unknown. However, factors that may be associated with hairy tongue include emotional stress, smoking, poor oral hygiene, oxidizing mouthwashes, radiation, systemic antibiotics, in particular, metronidazole, and *Candida albicans*.

Main Clinical Features

- Elongation of the filiform papillae of the tongue presenting as hair-like projections
- The filiform papillae may be yellowish-white, brown, or black in color
- Usually asymptomatic although some patients may complain of bad taste, a gagging sensation, or bad breath
- Appearance of the tongue may cause significant distress to the patients

Diagnosis

The diagnosis is exclusively based on the clinical features.

Differential Diagnosis

- Acanthosis nigricans
- Furred tongue
- Candidiasis

Treatment

Basic Guidelines

- Stop any predisposing etiologic factor.
- High level of oral hygiene.
- Patients should be reassured that the condition is benign.
- Recurrences are common.

Suggested Therapies

- In mild cases, brushing the dorsum of the tongue with a tongue cleaner every morning for 1 month or more may improve the condition.
- In severe cases, with very long filiform papillae, topical application of keratolytic agents such as 30–50% trichloroacetic acid or salicylic acid in alcohol or 40% urea in water destroys the elongated papillae and restores the tongue to normal. Trichloroacetic acid is the best and should be applied with care once. It can be reapplied in 1 week's time if there are remnants of the elongated papillae.
- Topical or systemic antifungals do not have no place in the treatment of hairy tongue.

References

Darwazeh AM, Pillai K. Prevalence of tongue lesions in 1013 Jordanian dental outpatients. *Comm Dent Oral Epidemiol* 1993;21:323–324.
Heymann WR. Psychotropic agent-induced black hairy tongue. *Cutis* 2000;66:25–26.
Laskaris G. *Color Atlas of Oral Diseases*, 3rd edition. Thieme Verlag: Stuttgart, 2003.

Hand, Foot, and Mouth Disease

Definition

Hand, foot, and mouth disease is an acute, endemic viral infection.

Etiology

The causative organisms are the coxsackievirus A16, A5, and A10.

Main Clinical Features

The disease usually affects children and young adults and may occur in epidemics or as isolated cases.

Oral Lesions

- A few (5–20) small vesicles that soon rupture, leaving slightly painful, shallow ulcers surrounded by a red halo
- Buccal mucosa, tongue, and palate are most frequently affected

Skin

- Small vesicles with a narrow red halo
- Lateral and dorsal surfaces of the fingers and toes, palms, soles, and buttocks are the sites of predilection

Constitutional Symptoms

- Low grade fever for 2–3 days
- Malaise
- Disease lasts 5–8 days

Diagnosis

The diagnosis is based on clinical criteria.

Differential Diagnosis

- Aphthous ulcers
- Herpetiform ulcers
- Primary herpetic gingivostomatitis
- Secondary herpes
- Herpangina

Treatment

- The treatment is symptomatic. Affected children should stay in bed for 3–4 days.
- There is no specific antiviral therapy. The role of acyclovir is debatable.
- Antipyretics, e. g., aspirin, for 4–6 days.
- Soft foods.
- The disease is self-limiting.

References

Faulkner CF, Godbolt AM, De Ambrosis B, Triscott I. Hand, foot and mouth disease in an immunocompromised adult treated with aciclovir. *Australas J Dermatol* 2003;44:203–206.

Frydenberg A, Starr M. Hand, foot and mouth disease. *Aust Fam Phys* 2003;32:594–595.

Laskaris G. Oral manifestations of infectious diseases. *Dent Clin North Am* 1996;40:395–423.

Shelley WB, Hashim M, Shelley ED. Acyclovir in the treatment of hand-foot-and-mouth disease. *Cutis* 1996;57: 232–234.

Tokutake T, Matsumiya C, Honjo A, Kato T. Hand, foot and mouth disease. *Nippon Rinsho* 2003;61(suppl 2):190–194.

Herpangina

Definition

Herpangina is an acute viral infection of the oral cavity.

Etiology

Coxsackievirus group A types 1–6, 8, 10, 12, 22 are the causative organisms. Recently, enterovirus 71 has also been found to be associated with herpangina.

Main Clinical Features

- Sudden fever (38–40 °C)
- Headache, malaise
- Sore throat, dysphagia
- Diffuse erythema and multiple vesicle formation in the oropharynx, soft palate, and uvula
- Vesicles soon rupture leaving painful, shallow, round ulcers
- Ulcers heal spontaneously in 7–10 days

Diagnosis

The diagnosis is based on clinical criteria.

Differential Diagnosis

- Primary herpetic gingivostomatitis
- Aphthous ulcers
- FAPA syndrome
- Acute lymphonodular pharyngitis
- Gonococcal oropharyngitis
- Streptococcal pharyngitis
- Erythema multiforme
- Hand, foot, and mouth disease

Treatment

- Corticosteroids in low doses, e. g., prednisone 10–20 mg/day, for 4–6 days, reduce the inflammation and pain dramatically.
- Analgesics for 3–6 days.
- Local use of antiseptic mouthwashes has limited usefulness.
- Soft foods are recommended.

References

Lang SD, Singh K. The sore throat. When to investigate and when to prescribe. *Drugs* 1990;40:854–862.

Laskaris G. Oral manifestations of infectious diseases. *Dent Clin North Am* 1996;40:395–423.

Lin TY, Chang LY, Hsia SH, et al. The 1998 enterovirus 71 outbreak in Taiwan: Pathogenesis and management. *Clin Infect Dis* 2002;34(suppl 2):552–557.

Urashima M, Shindo N, Okabe N. Seasonal models of herpangina and hand-foot-mouth disease to simulate annual fluctuations in urban warming in Tokyo. *Jpn J Infect Dis* 2003;56:48–53.

Waldfahrer F, Iro H. Successful treatment of herpangina with allopurinol mouthwashes. *Laryngoscope* 1995; 105:1405.

Herpes Simplex Virus Infections

■ Definition

Herpes simplex virus (HSV) is the most common herpetic infection of the oral and maxillofacial area.

■ Etiology

Herpesvirus type 1 and rarely type 2 are the causative organisms.

■ Classification

HSV infections are classified as primary (acute herpetic gingivostomatitis) and secondary (herpetic stomatitis, herpes labialis). Primary herpetic gingivostomatitis is mostly encountered in children and young adults whereas secondary herpetic stomatitis affects adults. Immunocompromised patients often present with recurrent, persistent intraoral herpetic lesions.

■ Main Clinical Features

Primary Herpetic Gingivostomatitis

Prodromal symptoms: High fever, irritability, malaise, headache, sore mouth, and painful cervical lymphadenopathy
Lesions: Multiple, small vesicles that rupture leaving round, shallow coalescing ulcers
Location: Gingiva, tongue, lips, palate, and buccal mucosa
Duration: 10–14 days

Secondary Herpetic Stomatitis

Prodromal symptoms: No constitutional symptoms
Lesions: Smaller and fewer lesions
Location: Hard palate and attached gingiva, pharyngotonsillar area
Duration: 6–10 days

Herpes Labialis

Prodromal symptoms: Burning, itching, and mild pain in the affected area lasting a few hours before the eruption

Lesions: Small clustering vesicles that rupture leaving ulcers that crust
Location: Vermillion border of the lip and perioral skin
Duration: 5–8 days

■ Diagnosis

The diagnosis is based on the clinical presentation. The definitive criterion for diagnosing a herpetic infection is isolation of the virus in tissue culture inoculated with the vesicular fluid.

■ Differential Diagnosis

- Aphthous ulcers
- Herpangina
- Hand, foot, and mouth disease
- Acute necrotizing ulcerative gingivitis
- Pemphigoid
- Erythema multiforme
- Pemphigus
- Streptococcal stomatitis
- Gonococcal stomatitis
- Primary and secondary syphilis
- Traumatic lesions

■ Treatment

Basic Guidelines

- Management of HSV-1 infections of the oral and perioral area is mostly palliative. It is important to assess the following factors when selecting the treatment modality:
  — the number of recurrences and whether the patient can perceive the prodromal symptoms early enough to initiate treatment
  — the patient's immune status.
- Systemic antiviral treatment is employed if the patient is immunocompromised or as a prophylactic regimen in patients who have frequent recurrences due to known trigger factors.
- Systemic antiviral agents should be used with caution.

- Patients should stay in bed for 4–6 days in cases of primary herpetic gingivostomatitis.
- Avoidance of spicy and hard foods and toothbrushing during the acute stage is recommended.

Suggested Therapies

Topical Treatment

Primary Herpetic Gingivostomatitis

Topical rinsing with 0.5 or 1% dyclonine hydrochloride is recommended for temporary relief.

Herpes Labialis

- Apply 5% acyclovir cream in a liposome carrier in the prodromal stage.
- 1.8% Tetracaine cream can be applied up to six times daily.

Systemic Treatment

Primary Herpetic Gingivostomatitis

- Acyclovir suspension 15 mg/kg or acyclovir tablets 200 mg five times daily for 5 days initiated in the first 3 days of onset can shorten the duration of the lesions.
- Acyclovir 800 mg daily may be used as a prophylactic regimen for as long as the symptom-free period usually lasts. If the patient is immunocompromised, higher doses with close monitoring may be required.
- Valacyclovir tablets 500 mg or famciclovir 250 mg twice daily for 5 days may be used as an alternative therapeutic regimen. This treatment is safe and effective.

References

Blevins JY. Primary herpetic gingivostomatitis in young children. *Pediatr Nurs* 2003;29:199–202.

Chauvin PJ, Ajar AH. Acute herpetic gingivostomatitis in adults: a review of 13 cases, including diagnosis and management. *J Can Dent Assoc* 2002;68:247–251.

Emmert DH. Treatment of common cutaneous herpes simplex virus infections. *Am Fam Phys* 2000;61:1697–1706.

Epstein JB, Ransier A, Sherlock CH, Spinelli JJ, Reece D. Acyclovir prophylaxis of oral herpes virus during bone marrow transplantation. *Eur J Cancer B Oral Oncol* 1996;32B:158–162.

Kaminester LH, Pariser RJ, Pariser DM, et al. A double-blind, placebo-controlled study of topical tetracaine in the treatment of herpes labialis. *J Am Acad Dermatol* 1999;41:996–1001.

Kiderman A, Furst AL, Miller T, et al. How successfully do general practitioners diagnose herpetic gingivostomatitis clinically? *Br J Gen Pract* 2002;52:481–482.

Spruance SL, McKeough MB. Combination treatment with famciclovir and a topical corticosteroid gel versus famciclovir alone for experimental ultraviolet radiation-induced herpes simplex labialis: A pilot study. *J Infect Dis* 2000;181:1906–1910.

Wu FF, Brentjens MH, Torres G, et al. Valacyclovir in the treatment of herpes simplex, herpes zoster, and other viral infections. *J Cutan Med Surg* 2003;7:372–381.

Herpes Zoster

▣ Definition

Herpes zoster or shingles is an acute inflammatory viral disease.

▣ Etiology

The causative organism is varicella-zoster virus (human herpesvirus 3).

▣ Main Clinical Features

The thoracic, cervical, trigeminal, and lumbosacral dermatomes are most frequently affected. Oral lesions occur if the second and third branches of the trigeminal nerve are involved.

Oral Lesions

- Itching sensation and pain, which may simulate pulpitis
- Unilateral cluster of vesicles which rupture in 2–3 days, leaving painful ulcers surrounded by a red zone
- Ulcers heal in 2–3 weeks
- Postherpetic trigeminal neuralgia and osteomyelitis of the jaw bone are the most common complication

Skin Lesions

- Intense pain associated with pruritus, tingling, and tenderness
- Painful eruption of vesicles on erythematous bases which develop along a sensory dermatome
- Rash typically involves a single dermatome and does not cross the midline but may involve multiple dermatomes
- Postherpetic neuralgia in 10–15% of cases

Constitutional Symptoms

- Fever
- Malaise
- Headache

▣ Diagnosis

The diagnosis is usually made clinically but may be aided by culture, direct fluorescent antibody test, serology and PCR.

▣ Differential Diagnosis

- Herpetic gingivostomatitis
- Necrotizing ulcerative gingivitis
- Varicella
- Erythema multiforme

▣ Treatment

Basic Guidelines

- Patients should be isolated and stay in bed for 1 week.
- The diagnosis should be made and treatment begun as early as possible.
- Immunocompromised patients must be hospitalized.

Suggested Therapies

- Antivirals
    - Valacyclovir 1 g three times daily for 7 days and famciclovir 500 mg three times daily for 7 days are the drugs of choice because of the more convenient dose regimens than acyclovir.
    - Traditionally, oral acyclovir 800 mg five times daily for 7–10 days has been used in the treatment of herpes zoster. High-dose i. v. acyclovir (30 mg/kg per day) for at least 7 days is recommended for the treatment of herpes zoster in immunocompromised patients.
- Analgesics, tranquilizers, tricyclic antidepressants, antiepileptics (carbamazepine, gabapentin) have been used for pain relief.
- Corticosteroids
    - Early use of prednisone 20–30 mg/day for 7–10 days tapered to 10 mg/day for 1 week has been used to reduce the incidence of postherpetic neuralgia in elderly patients. Corticosteroids must be avoided in immunocompromised patients.

References

Colgan R, Michocki R, Greisman L, Moore TA. Antiviral drugs in the immunocompetent host: Part I. Treatment of hepatitis, cytomegalovirus, and herpes infections. *Am Fam Phys* 2003;67:757–762.

Gross G, Schofer H, Wassilew S, et al. Herpes zoster guideline of the German Dermatology Society. *J Clin Virol* 2003;26:277–289.

Nikkels AF, Pierard GE. Oral antivirals revisited in the treatment of herpes zoster: What do they accomplish? *Am J Clin Dermatol* 2002;3:591–598.

Santee JA. Corticosteroids for herpes zoster: What do they accomplish? *Am J Clin Dermatol* 2002;3:517–524.

Wu JJ, Brentjens MH, Torres G, et al. Valacyclovir in the treatment of herpes simplex, herpes zoster, and other viral infections. *J Cutan Med Surg* 2003;7:372–381.

Histoplasmosis

■ Definition

Histoplasmosis is a systemic fungal disease endemic in the North and South Americas and may be found in other areas including Central America and certain parts of Africa and Asia. Sporadic cases have also been reported in Europe.

■ Etiology

Histoplasmosis is caused by *Histoplasma capsulatum*, a dimorphic fungus. The organism is found in humid climates and grows readily in soil containing bird or bat excrement. The disease is acquired by inhaling the microconidia or small spores.

■ Classification

There are three major forms of symptomatic histoplasmosis: a) acute pulmonary, b) chronic pulmonary, and c) disseminated.

■ Main Clinical Features

Infection is common in endemic areas but is often asymptomatic or results in a self-limiting undiagnosed illness. The oral mucosa is affected in about 35–45% of cases of the disseminated form. Rarely the oral lesions may be the initial or the only manifestation of the disease.

Acute Pulmonary Histoplasmosis

This is the most common form and is characterized by chest pain and cough, lymphadenopathy and constitutional symptoms (low-grade fever, malaise, chills, myalgias). It is not associated with oral lesions.

Chronic Pulmonary Histoplasmosis

This form is characterized by progressive infiltration, cavitation, and scarring and occurs in individuals with underlying pulmonary disease. It is not associated with oral lesions.

Disseminated Histoplasmosis

The disseminated form represents about 10% of the symptomatic cases of histoplasmosis. It is a progressive illness with fever and weight loss and commonly occurs in individuals with underlying immunosuppressive disorders such as HIV infection. The infection involves the bone marrow, liver, spleen, gastrointestinal tract, adrenal glands, central nervous system, and skin and mucosal surfaces. Clinically, oral lesions present as indurated, painful ulcers or verrucous, nodular, or granulomatous lesions.

■ Diagnosis

Histoplasmosis is diagnosed by biopsy and histopathologic examination, culture, and serologic tests for antibodies or polysaccharide antigen. Chest radiograph is also necessary.

■ Differential Diagnosis

- Blastomycosis
- Coccidioidomycosis
- Paracoccidioidomycosis
- Cryptococcosis
- Aspergillosis
- Mucormycosis
- Leishmaniasis
- Squamous cell carcinoma
- Tuberculosis
- Non-Hodgkin lymphoma
- Malignant granuloma
- Wegener granulomatosis
- Necrotizing sialadenometaplasia

■ Treatment

Basic Guidelines

- Histoplasmosis must be treated by the specialist.
- The role of the oral physician (stomatologist) is limited to diagnosis of oral histoplasmosis or to the treatment of localized oral histoplasmosis but in collaboration with the specialist.
- The treatment is always systemic.

Suggested Therapies

Itraconazole is the most effective triazole against *H. capsulatum.* An initial dose of 200 mg three times per day for 3–4 days is recommended. The dose is later limited to 200–400 mg/day for 6–12 weeks for the acute pulmonary form and for 12–24 months in patients with chronic pulmonary form. For disseminated histoplasmosis itraconazole 200–400 mg/day is given for about 6–16 months or more. For localized oral lesions itraconazole 200 mg/day for 2–3 months is recommended. Itraconazole is as effective as amphotericin B and ketoconazole but is better tolerated than either. Side effects and interactions with other drugs must be taken into consideration during treatment with itraconazole.

Ketoconazole 400 mg/day is the drug of second choice for oral treatment of histoplasmosis and given for weeks to several months depending on the form and severity of the disease. Ketoconazole is less active and less well tolerated than itraconazole.

Amphotericin B is very effective and is reserved for patients with severe illness or patients who cannot take oral drugs or have failed to respond to itraconazole. Fungizone or the newer types of amphotericin (AmBisome, Abelcet, Amphotec) may be used intravenously. However, because of the severe side effects, amphotericin therapy must be given only by specialists in a hospital unit.

Corticosteroids, e.g., prednisone 30–40 mg/day, can be used for 2–3 weeks to alleviate the pulmonary symptoms but should always be given in combination with the antifungal therapy.

Future Therapies

The newer third generation triazoles (voriconazole, posaconazole, ravuconazole, and others) and the echinocandins or pneumocandins may provide alternatives to the current antifungals for the treatment of systemic mycoses.

References

Couppie P, Clyti E, Nacher M, et al. Acquired immunodeficiency syndrome-related oral and/or cutaneous histoplasmosis: A descriptive and comparative study of 21 cases in French Guiana. *Int J Dermatol* 2002;41:571–576.

Dismukes WE. Introduction of antifungal drugs. *Clin Infect Dis* 2000;30:653–657.

Ferreira OG, Cardoso SV, Boerges AS, et al. Oral histoplasmosis in Brasil. *Oral Surg Oral Med Oral Pathol Oral Radiol Endod* 2002;93:654–659.

Letscher-Bru V, Herbecht R. Caspofungin: The first representative of a new antifungal class. *J Antimicrob Chemother* 2003;51:513–521.

Pierard GE, Arrese JE, Pierrard-Franchimont C. Itraconazole. *Expert Clin Pharmacother* 2000;1:287–304.

Stevens DA. New directions in antifungal therapy. *Jpn J Med Mycol* 1997;38:141–144.

Terrell GL. Antifungal agents. Part II. The azoles. *Mayo Clin Proc* 1999;74:78–100.

Infectious Mononucleosis

Definition

Infectious mononucleosis is an acute self-limiting infectious disease.

Etiology

The causative organism is the Epstein–Barr virus (human herpesvirus 4).

Main Clinical Features

The disease is more common in children and young adults. The oral lesions are relatively common.

Oral Mucosa

- Palatal petechiae
- Diffuse erythema
- Uvular edema
- Gingivitis
- Ulcers, rarely
- Sore throat
- Tonsillar exudate
- Tonsillitis
- Pharyngitis

Skin

- Maculopapular eruption
- Petechial rash

Constitutional Signs and Symptoms

- Fever
- Malaise, anorexia, myalgia
- Lymphadenopathy
- Splenomegaly
- Liver involvement
- CNS involvement
- Renal and pulmonary involvement
- Myocarditis

Diagnosis

The diagnosis should be confirmed by the monospot test and heterophil antibody test.

Differential Diagnosis

- Diphtheria
- Gonococcal stomatitis
- Streptococcal infections
- Herpes simplex
- Herpangina
- Secondary syphilis
- Leukemia
- Fellatio

Treatment

Basic Guidelines

- The patient should stay in bed for about 1 week.
- The treatment is symptomatic.
- The treatment must be carried out by a specialist.

Suggested Therapies

- Symptomatic relief can be achieved by the administration of nonsteroidal anti-inflammatory agents.
- Aspirin or acetaminophen may also be used.
- Warm saline gargles three to four times daily.
- Corticosteroids in low doses, e.g., prednisone 20 mg/day, in a 10-day tapering course should be reserved for complicated cases.
- Antiviral agents are usually not helpful.

References

Chalres PG. Infectious mononucleosis. *Aust Fam Phys* 2003;32:785–788.

Goldani LZ. Treatment of severe infectious mononucleosis with famciclovir. *J Infect* 2002;44:92–93.

Lekstrom-Himes JA, Dale JK, Kingma DW, Diaz PS, Jaffe ES, Straus SE. Periodic illness associated with Epstein–Barr virus infection. *Clin Infect Dis* 1996;22:22.

Murray PG, Young LS. Epstein–Barr virus infection: Basis of malignancy and potential for therapy. *Expert Rev Mol Med* 2001;15:1–20.

Infectious Sialadenitis

Definition

Infectious sialadenitis is a relatively common, acute infectious disease of the major salivary glands.

Etiology

Staphylococcus aureus, S. pyogenes, Streptococcus viridans and other bacteria of the oral flora may be the causative organisms.

Main Clinical Features

- Painful swelling
- Induration
- Inflammation and pus discharge from the duct opening
- Overlying skin may be red and tense
- Low-grade fever
- Malaise

Diagnosis

The diagnosis is usually made on clinical criteria. Gram stain and culture may be helpful.

Differential Diagnosis

- Mumps
- Obstructive sialadenitis
- Sjögren syndrome
- Mikulicz syndrome
- Heerfordt syndrome
- Non-Hodgkin lymphoma
- Hodgkin lymphoma
- Lymph node enlargement
- Salivary gland neoplasms

Treatment

Basic Guidelines

- Maintenance of good oral hygiene.
- Adequate hydration.

Suggested Therapies

- Oral dicloxacillin 250–500 mg every 8 hours for 6–8 days or flucloxacillin 250–500 mg every 8 hours for 6–8 days is recommended.
- Oral cephalosporins such as cephalexin 250–500 mg every 8 hours for 6–8 days may also be used.
- Oral macrolides such as erythromycin 250–500 mg every 8 hours for 6–10 days may also be used.

References

Brook I. Acute bacterial suppurative parotitis: Microbiology and management. *J Craniofac Surg* 2003;14:37–40.

Curtin-Wirt C, Casey JR, Murray PC, et al. Efficacy of penicillin vs amoxicillin in children with group A hemolytic streptococcal tonsillopharyngitis. *Clin Pediatr* 2003;42:219–225.

Laskaris G. *Color Atlas of Oral Diseases*, 3rd edition. Thieme Verlag: Stuttgart, 2003.

Kawasaki Syndrome

■ Definition

Kawasaki syndrome or mucocutaneous lymph node syndrome is an acute multisystem vasculitis of infancy and childhood.

■ Etiology

The etiology is unknown. However, it is thought that *Staphylococcus aureus* superantigens may trigger the disease.

■ Main Clinical Features

The oral manifestations of Kawasaki disease are relatively common.

Oral Lesions

- Erythema, edema, and fissuring of the lips
- Enlarged and red tongue papillae
- Deep red palate and oropharynx
- Rarely ulcers

Skin Lesions

- Erythema and edema of hands and feet following by peeling, usually of the tips of the fingers and toes
- Polymorphous nonvesicular skin rash

Other Symptoms and Signs

- Conjunctivitis, uveitis
- Arthralgia, arthritis
- Abdominal symptoms
- Cardiovascular disorders
- Encephalitis
- Renal involvement
- Coronary artery involvement

Constitutional Symptoms

- Fever (38.3–40 °C) lasting for at least 5 days
- Malaise, anorexia
- Cervical lymphadenopathy

■ Diagnosis

The diagnosis is based on clinical criteria.

■ Differential Diagnosis

- Scarlet fever
- Erythema multiforme
- Staphylococcal scalded skin syndrome
- Herpetic gingivostomatitis

■ Treatment

Basic Guidelines

- Early diagnosis and treatment shorten the course of the disease.
- Treatment of oral lesions is part of the systemic treatment.
- The management should be undertaken by a pediatrician.

Suggested Therapies

- Aspirin 80–100 mg/kg per day in four divided doses with subsequent tapering over 6–10 weeks along with i.v. immunoglobulin 2 g/kg over 12 hours is the mainstay of treatment.
- Corticosteroids, in addition to i.v. immunoglobulin therapy, may be used in the acute phase of Kawasaki disease.
- Plasmapheresis may be useful in cases that do not respond to immunoglobulin treatment.

References

Gedalia A. Kawasaki disease: An update. *Curr Rheumatol Rep* 2002;4:25–29.

Jacobs JC. Kawasaki disease. *Curr Opin Rheumatol* 1996;8: 41–47.

Lang B, Duffy CM. Controversies in the management of Kawasaki disease. *Best Pract Res Clin Rheumatol* 2002;16: 427–442.

Leung DY. The potential role of bacterial superantigens in the pathogenesis of Kawasaki syndrome. *J Clin Immunol* 1995;15:115.

Sundel RP, Baker AL, Fulton DR, Newburger JW. Corticosteroids in the initial treatment of Kawasaki disease: A randomized trial. *J Pediatr* 2003;142:611–616.

Langerhans Cell Histiocytosis

▓ Definition

Langerhans cell histiocytosis or histiocytosis-X is a clonal proliferative disease of the Langerhans cells.

▓ Etiology

The etiology is unknown. A genetic predisposition in association with viral infection and immunologic mechanisms are possibly involved in the pathogenesis of the disease.

▓ Classification

The disease spectrum includes four types: a) Letterer–Siwe disease, b) Hand–Schüller–Christian disease, c) eosinophilic granuloma, and d) Hashimoto–Pritzker disease or congenital Langerhans cell histiocytosis.

▓ Main Clinical Features

Oral lesions may occur in all four types.

Letterer–Siwe Disease

- Acute multisystemic form which appears during the first year of life
- Oral lesions are relatively common, presenting as ulcers, ecchymosis, gingivitis, periodontitis, and loose teeth
- Skin rash (papules, pustules, vesicles, petechiae, purpura, scales and crusts) is common
- Lung, liver, bone, lymph nodes, and the hematopoietic system are commonly involved
- Prognosis is poor

Hand–Schüller–Christian Disease

- Chronic disseminated form which manifests between 3 and 6 years
- Classic triad of the disease consists of bone lesions, diabetes insipidus, and exophthalmos
- Oral lesions are common and present as ulcers, edema, gingivitis, jaw bone involvement, severe periodontitis, and tooth loss
- Skin lesions and otitis media are common
- Prognosis is usually good

Eosinophilic Granuloma

- Localized form which usually affects adolescents
- Asymptomatic osteolytic bones lesions are the most common manifestations
- Jaw bones may be affected leading to bone destruction and tooth loss
- Oral mucosal ulcers may also occur
- Prognosis is good

Hashimoto–Pritzker Disease

- Congenital self-healing form
- Disease begins at birth or in the first days of life
- Lesions are limited to the skin (red to brown nodules, crusts, papules, vesicles)
- Oral mucosa is rarely affected
- Prognosis is excellent

▓ Diagnosis

The diagnosis should be confirmed by biopsy and histopathologic examination, radiographs, and immunohistochemical examination.

▓ Differential Diagnosis

- Eosinophilic ulcer
- Aggressive periodontitis
- Necrotizing ulcerative gingivitis and periodontitis
- Hypophosphatasia
- Acatalasia
- Leukemia
- Multiple myeloma

▨ Treatment

Basic Guidelines

- The role of the oral clinician is limited to the treatment of the oral manifestations of this group of diseases.
- A follow-up program is necessary as recurrences are common.
- The systemic treatment must be carried out by a specialist.

Suggested Therapies

- Localized oral lesions (eosinophilic granuloma, bone, and oral mucosa) may be treated successfully with surgical curettage or excision. Intralesional corticosteroid injections or a low-dose regimen of systemic oral corticosteroids, e. g., prednisone 20–30 mg/day for 2–4 weeks and then tapering the dose may also be useful. Low-dose radiation is an alternative procedure for localized bone lesions.
- Multisystemic disease (Letterer–Siwe and Hand–Schüller–Christian disease) needs systemic chemotherapy. The most common agents used in different combination regimens and several cycles are corticosteroids, vinblastine, etoposide, cytarabine, 6-mercaptopurine, methotrexate, 2-chlorodeoxyadenosine, cyclosporine, thalidomide, and others.

References

Arico M, Girschikofsky M, Genereau T, et al. Langerhans cell histiocytosis in adults. Report from the International Registry of the Histiocyte Society. *Eur J Cancer* 2003;39:2341–2348.

Broadbent V, Gadner H. Current therapy for Langerhans cell histiocytosis. *Hematol Oncol Clin North Am* 1998;12:327–338.

Eckardt A, Schultze A. Maxillofacial manifestations of Langerhans cell histiocytosis: A clinical and therapeutic analysis of 10 patients. *Oral Oncol* 2003;39:687–694.

Goh NS, McDonald CE, McGregor DP, et al. Successful treatment of Langerhans cell histiocytosis with 2-chlorodeoxyadenosine. *Respirology* 2003;8:91–94.

Pardanani A, Phyliky RL, Li CY, Tefferi A. 2-chlorodeoxyadenosine therapy for disseminated Langerhans cell histiocytosis. *Mayo Clin Proc* 2003;78:301–306.

Willman CL, Busque L, Griffith BB, et al. Langerhans cell histiocytosis (histiocytosis-X): A clonal proliferative disease. *N Engl J Med* 1994;331:154–160.

Leishmaniasis

Definition

Leishmaniasis is a relatively common protozoan disease. It is endemic in the Mediterranean countries, South America, and areas of Africa and Asia.

Etiology

Leishmaniasis is caused by parasites of the genus *Leishmania*. Sandflies from the genus *Phlebotomus* transfer the parasite from infected animals to humans.

Classification

There are three forms of the disease: a) cutaneous leishmaniasis caused by *L. tropica*, b) mucocutaneous leishmaniasis caused by *L. brasiliensis*, and c) systemic or visceral leishmaniasis (Kala-azar) caused by *L. donovani*.

Main Clinical Features

The oral lesions are rare and may develop as part of cutaneous or mucocutaneous leishmaniasis.

Oral Lesions

The oral lesions usually present as red nodules or plaques that progressively enlarge leading to ulceration. In severe mucocutaneous leishmaniasis, perforation of the palate may occur. The lips are the sites of predilection, following by the palate, buccal mucosa, and gingiva

Skin Lesions

Cutaneous leishmaniasis usually begins as a small well-demarcated papule that progressively enlarges into a nodule or plaque, which may become ulcerated. The face, neck, arms, and legs are more frequently affected. The lesions are usually solitary but may be multiple

Diagnosis

The diagnosis is based on biopsy and histopathologic examination. *Leishmania* skin test and serologic tests may also be useful.

Differential Diagnosis

- Basal cell carcinoma
- Squamous cell carcinoma
- Keratoacanthoma
- Non-Hodgkin lymphoma
- Wegener granulomatosis
- Malignant granuloma
- Systemic mycoses
- Staphylococcal infection
- Syphilis
- Sarcoidosis
- Discoid lupus erythematosus

Treatment

Basic Guidelines

- Prevention of leishmaniasis should be the target.
- Treatment depends upon the clinical form and the severity of the disease.
- The oral lesions should usually be treated as part of cutaneous leishmaniasis.
- The course of the disease is dependent on host immunity and the species of the parasite.

Suggested Therapies

Systemic Treatment

- Meglumine antimonate 20–30 mg/kg per day, i.v. or i.m. for 3–4 weeks is the drug of choice. Side effects of the drug must always be borne in mind.
- Sodium stibogluconate 20 mg/kg per day for 3 weeks is also recommended for more severe cases.

Topical Treatment

Intralesional sodium stibogluconate 0.2–0.4 ml three times a week for a total of 5 weeks is usually effective; 20 % paromomycin sulfate is an alternative topical treatment. Surgical excision, CO_2 laser, and cryotherapy have also a place in the therapeutic armamentarium.

Alternative Therapies

Alternative systemic therapies of cutaneous and mucocutaneous forms of leishmaniasis include itraconazole, ketoconazole, amphotericin B, allopurinol, pentamidine, and interferon.

References

Berman JD. Current treatment approaches to leishmaniasis. *Curr Opin Infect Dis* 2003;16:397–401.

Chaudry Z, Barrett AW, Corbett E, et al. Oral mucosal leishmaniasis as a presenting feature of HIV infection and its management. *J Oral Pathol Med* 1999;28:43–48.

Herwaldt BL, Berman JD. Recommendations for treating leishmaniasis with sodium stibogluconate (Pentostam) and review of pertinent clinical studies. *Am J Trop Med Hyg* 1992;46:296.

Kolde G, Luger T, Sorg C, et al. Successful treatment of cutaneous leishmaniasis using systemic interferon gamma. *Dermatology* 1996;192:56–60.

Lee SA, Hasbun R. Therapy of cutaneous leishmaniasis. *Int J Infect Dis* 2003;86–93.

Sangueza OP, Sungueza JM, et al. Mucocutaneous leishmaniasis: A clinicopathologic classification. *J Am Acad Dermatol* 1993;28:927–932.

Sitheeque MAM, Qazi AA, Ahmed GA. A study of cutaneous leishmaniasis involvement of the lips and perioral tissues. *Br J Oral Maxillofac Surg* 1990;28:43–48.

Uzun S, Uslular C, Yücel A, et al. Cutaneous leishmaniasis: Evaluation of 3074 cases in the Cukurova region of Turkey. *Br J Dermatol* 1999;140:347–350.

Leukemias

▓ Definition

Leukemias are a heterogeneous group of hematological malignant disorders that originate from hematopoietic stem cells and are characterized by a defect in the maturation and proliferation of leukocytes.

▓ Etiology

Leukemias are probably the result of a combination of genetic and environmental factors.

▓ Classification

Leukemias are classified according to their origin and histogenetic criteria as myelocytic and lymphocytic, and according to their clinical presentation as acute and chronic.

▓ Main Clinical Features

Oral manifestations have been recorded in 30–80 % of patients with leukemia and are more frequently seen in acute rather than in chronic leukemia.

Oral Lesions

- Mucosal pallor, petechiae, ecchymoses. and bleeding
- Oral ulcerations, gingival enlargement, tooth mobility
- Delayed wound healing, laryngeal pain, cervical and submandibular lymphadenopathy
- Bacterial, viral, and mycotic infections are common oral complications
- Poor oral hygiene may predispose the patients to develop oral lesions

Systemic Manifestations

- Fever, chills, weakness, fatigue, weight loss, headache
- Skin pallor, bleeding, bone pain
- Hepatosplenomegaly
- Generalized lymphadenopathy

▓ Diagnosis

The clinical diagnosis should be confirmed by oral biopsy, blood count, bone marrow biopsy, and histochemical and immunological tests.

▓ Differential Diagnosis

- Neutropenia
- Cyclic neutropenia
- Agranulocytosis
- Aplastic anemia
- Thrombocytopenic purpura
- Myelodysplastic syndromes
- Non-Hodgkin lymphoma
- Hodgkin lymphoma
- Gingival fibromatosis
- Gingival enlargement due to drugs

▓ Treatment

Basic Guidelines

- High level of oral hygiene.
- Antibacterial rinses, e.g., chlorhexidine and hydrogen peroxide may be used prophylactically.
- Bacterial, viral, and fungal oral infections should be treated as soon as possible.
- The oral lesions usually regress during the systemic treatment of leukemia.
- The systemic treatment must be carried out by a specialist hematologist.

Suggested Therapies

Topical Treatment

- Topical application of 0.1 % triamcinolone acetonide in Orabase, or clobetasol gel, or tacrolimus paste two to four times daily improves the symptoms and helps the lesions to heal.
- 1 % povidone iodine solution may also be used.

Systemic Treatment

Supportive Therapy

Supportive therapy includes red cell and platelet transfusion, granulocyte colony-stimulating factor (G-CSF), recombinant erythropoietin administration etc, depending on the status of the disease and the needs of the patient.

Antileukemic Therapy

- *Chronic leukemias*: For chronic B-lymphocytic leukemia, oral chlorambucil is effective. In the past decade i.v. or oral fludarabine administration has also been shown to be highly effective. For chronic myelocytic leukemia, hydroxyurea orally combined with s.c. interferon alpha had proved to be very effective. However, in the past few years imatinib mesylate (Gleevec), a tyrosine kinase inhibitor, has been used with excellent results and negligible toxicity.
- *Acute leukemias*: For acute lymphocytic leukemia, combination chemotherapy including corticosteroids is used. The drugs of choice for this type of protocol are vincristine, daunorubicin, cyclophosphamide, methotrexate, and asparaginase. The acute nonlymphocytic leukemias are usually treated with a combination of daunorubicin and cytosine arabinoside. If complete remission is achieved, depending on the patient's age and availability of a compatible donor, consolidation therapy with allogenic stem cell transplantation is used. For acute promyelocytic leukemia, the treatment is based on the administration of all-*trans* retinoic acid (ATRA), a differentiating factor in combination with daunorubicin. Cases of erythroleukemia may be treated either conservatively when the patient is elderly or similar to acute nonlymphoblastic leukemia.
  - Future treatment strategies for patients with acute myeloid leukemia most likely will include combinations of biologic agents with defined molecular targets, e. g., monoclonal antibodies, tyrosine kinase inhibitors, retinoids, and hypomethylating agents.

References

Cho SY, Cheng AC, Cheng MC. Oral care for children with leukemia. *Hong Kong Med J* 2000;6:203–208.

Hou GL, Huang JS, Tsai CC. Analysis of oral manifestations of leukemia: A retrospective study. *Oral Dis* 1997;3:31–38.

Iovino CS, Camacho LH. Acute myeloid leukemia: A classification and treatment update. *Clin J Oncol Nurs* 2003; 7:535–540.

Kantarjian H, O'Brien S, Cortes J, et al. Analysis of the impact of imatinib mesylate on the prognosis of patients with Philadelphia chromosome-positive chronic myelogenous leukemia treated with interferon-alpha regimens for early chronic phase. *Cancer* 2003;98:1430–1437.

Majorana A, Schubert MM, Porta F, et al. Oral complications of pediatric hematopoietic cell transplantation: diagnosis and management. *Support Care Cancer* 2000;8:353–365.

Ravandi F, Kantarjian H, Giles F, Cortes J. New agents in acute myeloid leukemia and other myeloid disorders. *Cancer* 2004;100:441–454.

Shanafelt TD, Call TG. Current approach to diagnosis and management of chronic lymphocytic leukemia. *Mayo Clin Proc* 2004;79:388–398.

Silver RT. Chronic myeloid leukemia. *Hematol Oncol Clin North Am* 2003;17:1159–1173.

Wu J, Fantasia JE, Kaplan R. Oral manifestations of acute myelomonocytic leukemia: A case report and review of the classification of leukemias. *J Periodontol* 2002;73: 664–668.

Leukoplakia

▓ Definition

Leukoplakia is a clinical term. It is a precancerous lesion, defined as a white patch or plaque of the oral mucosa that cannot be detached and cannot be identified as a lesion belonging to a specific disease entity.

▓ Etiology

The precise etiology of leukoplakia is still obscure. The main predisposing factors are smoking, alcohol, human papillomavirus (HPV), *Candida albicans*, and chronic trauma.

▓ Classification

There are three main clinical forms of oral leukoplakia: a) homogeneous, b) speckled, and c) proliferative verrucous.

▓ Main Clinical Features

Homogeneous

- White, asymptomatic, homogeneous plaque
- Surface is usually smooth or wrinkled and occasionally may be traversed by fissures or cracks
- Low risk for malignant transformation (2–4%)
- Most common form (92–96%)

Speckled

- Red background with multiple small white macules
- *C. albicans* infection is often present
- High risk for malignant transformation (20–30%)
- Rare

Proliferative Verrucous

- White exophytic papillary surface
- Tendency for prompt extension
- High risk for malignant transformation (30–40%)
- Very rare

▓ Diagnosis

Biopsy and histopathologic examination is the key to define the nature and the relative risk of leukoplakia. Molecular biological and immunohistochemical techniques (p53 antigen, HPV 16, 18, 33) are important for the detection of leukoplakia in cases with high risk for malignant transformation.

▓ Differential Diagnosis

- Lichen planus
- Discoid lupus erythematosus
- Candidiasis
- Hairy leukoplakia
- Cinnamon contact stomatitis
- Uremic stomatitis
- Leukoedema
- Chronic biting
- Chemical burn
- Several genetic diseases with oral keratinization

▓ Treatment

Basic Guidelines

- Improvement in oral hygiene.
- Elimination or discontinuation of all predisposing factors, specially smoking.
- Before any treatment a biopsy and histopathologic examination is always necessary to detect the presence or absence of epithelial dysplasia.
- Molecular biologic marker profile should be done.
- The size and the site of the lesions are important in the formulation of a treatment plan.
- A regular follow-up of patients with treated leukoplakia is mandatory for effective prevention of recurrence.

Suggested Therapies

- Surgical excision is the mainstay of the treatment of leukoplakia. Complete removal is suggested for a) homogeneous leukoplakia with epithelial dysplasia or without dysplasia but with p53 expression greater than baseline, b) speckled leukoplakia, and c) proliferative verrucous leukoplakia.

- Carbon dioxide (CO_2) laser surgery may be used as an alternative procedure.
- Cryosurgery and electrodessication are therapeutic modalities have limited results.
- In widespread or multiple leukoplakia oral administration of 13-*cis*-retinoic acid (1 mg/ kg body weight daily for 2–3 months) may be used with limited success. In addition, the severe side effects of the drugs further limit the utility of this approach.
- Topical application of retinoic acid (solution or in Orabase cream or in mucoadhesive slow-release two-layer tablets) has been used in the treatment of selective cases of leukoplakia with very limited success.
- Homogeneous leukoplakia without epithelial dysplasia may disappear or diminish in size within 2–3 months after the patient stops smoking, particularly if the lesion is located in the floor of the mouth.

Future Therapies

Photodynamic therapy using topically applied δ-aminolevulinic or 5-aminolevulinic acid.

References

Gaeta GM, Gombos F, Femiano F, et al. Acitretin and treatment of oral leukoplakia: A model for active molecule release. *J Eur Acad Dermatol Venereol* 2000;14:473–478.

Laskaris G. How to treat oral leukoplakia. *J Eur Acad Dermatol Venereol* 2000;14:446–447.

Scully C, Sudbo J, Speight PM. Progress in determining the malignant potential of oral lesions. *J Oral Pathol Med* 2003;32:251–256.

Sieron A, Adamec M, Mazur S, et al. Photodynamic therapy using topically applied -aminolevulinic acid for the treatment of oral leukoplakia. *J Oral Pathol Med* 2003; 32:330–336.

Thomson PJ, Wylie J. Interventional laser surgery: An effective surgical and diagnostic tool in oral precancer management. *Int J Oral Maxillofac Surg* 2002;31:145–153.

Van der Waal I, Axell T. Oral leukoplakia: A proposal for uniform reporting. *Oral Oncol* 2002;38:521–526.

Lichen Planus

▤ Definition

Lichen planus is a relatively common chronic inflammatory mucocutaneous disease.

▤ Etiology

Genetic, environmental, drug, and lifestyle factors may be involved in the pathogenesis of the disease. Cell-mediated immunity appears to play an important role in the pathogenesis of lichen planus.

▤ Main Clinical Features

Oral lichen planus is more common than the cutaneous type and oral lesions may occur independently of skin lesions. Polygonal white papules and lines are the basic clinical features of the diseases.

Oral Mucosa

Seven basic clinical forms of oral lichen planus have been described: *papular, reticular, erosive, atrophic, hypertrophic, bullous,* and *pigmented.* The buccal mucosa, tongue, lips, and gingiva are more frequently affected in a symmetrical pattern. Gingival lesions usually appear in the form of *desquamative gingivitis.* Most oral lesions are asymptomatic but erosive, atrophic, bullous, and gingival lesions may cause symptoms ranging from soreness to severe pain

Other Mucosae

The glans penis, vulva, and vagina may be involved

Skin

The skin lesions consist of slightly erythematous to violaceous pruritic papules usually on the flexor surfaces of the forearms and wrists, back and nails. Commonly, there is a symmetrical pattern

▤ Diagnosis

The diagnosis of lichen planus is usually based on the clinical criteria alone. In difficult cases the diagnosis should be confirmed by histopathologic examination and direct immunofluorescence.

▤ Differential Diagnosis

- Discoid lupus erythematosus
- Cicatricial pemphigoid
- Bullous pemphigoid
- Pemphigus
- Candidiasis
- Leukoplakia
- Chronic ulcerative stomatitis
- Cinnamon contact stomatitis
- Lichenoid reaction to dental restorative materials
- Graft-versus-host disease
- Plasma cell gingivitis
- Granulomatous gingivitis
- Psoriasis

▤ Treatment

Basic Guidelines

- Asymptomatic forms of oral lichen planus do not need therapy.
- Dental restorative materials such as amalgam and gold near the oral lesions should be replaced by other materials as they may produce lichenoid reactions or aggravate the lichen planus lesions.
- Composite restorations have also been implicated in oral lichenoid reactions.
- Stop tobacco and alcohol consumption.
- Treatment can be systemic or topical, depending on the form of the disease and the severity of the oral lesions.
- Recurrences after discontinuation of treatment are common.
- Very good oral hygiene should be maintained.
- The oral lesions may get infected with *Candida.*

Suggested Therapies

Systemic Treatment

Oral Corticosteroids

Oral corticosteroids (prednisone or prednisolone) 20–40 mg/day are the mainstay of treatment in severe, symptomatic oral lichen planus, particularly the erosive form. The lesions usually respond well in about 2–3 weeks and then the dose can be tapered to 5 mg every week and finally stopped not later than 4–6 weeks. The side effects of corticosteroids limit their use to topical preparations, particularly for long-term maintenance therapy. In addition, systemic corticosteroids should be avoided in hepatitis C-related oral lichen planus as they can increase HCV viremia.

Immunosuppressive Drugs

Azathioprine 50–100 mg/day and cyclosporine 3–5 mg/kg per day have been used with partial success as corticosteroid-sparing adjuncts to systemic corticosteroid therapy or as single-modality treatment if corticosteroid use is contraindicated. However, both immunosuppressive agents should be avoided in the treatment of oral lichen planus and used only in exceptional cases.

Retinoids

Systemic retinoids have no place in the treatment of oral lichen planus as complete remission is difficult to achieve and there is the possibility of severe adverse effects (teratogenicity, acute depression).

Other Drugs

Dapsone, levamisole, hydroxychloroquine sulfate, thalidomide, and pentoxifylline have been used but with doubtful results.

Topical Treatment

Topical corticosteroids applied in an adhesive paste (triamcinolone acetonide, fluocinolone acetonide, fluocinonide, clobetasol propionate) are usually effective and control the disease. They are particularly useful in maintaining the therapeutic result after systemic corticosteroid therapy. Intralesional injection of triamcinolone acetonide or betamethasone dipropionate and sodium phosphate in resistant localized erosions is effective.

Topical tacrolimus in a 0.5% adhesive ointment form appears to be effective in controlling erosive oral lichen planus. Topical mouth rinses of cyclosporine may also partially improve oral lesions.

Alternative Therapies

Systemic interferon alpha, glycyrrhizin, and photodynamic therapy may be useful in the future for treatment of oral lichen planus.

References

Carbone M, Controtto D, Carrozzo M, et al. Topical corticosteroids in association with miconazole and chlorhexidine in the long-term management of atrophic-erosive oral lichen planus: a placebo-controlled and comparative study between clobetasol and fluocinonide. *Oral Dis* 1999;5:41–49.

Carrozzo M, Gandolfo S. The management of oral lichen planus. *Oral Dis* 1999;5:196–205.

Jungell P, Malmstrom M. Cyclosporin A mouthwash in the treatment of oral lichen planus. *Int J Oral Maxillofac Surg* 1996;25:60–62.

Kaliakatsou F, Hodgson TA, Lewsey JD, et al. Management of recalcitrant ulcerative oral lichen planus with topical tacrolimus. *J Am Acad Dermatol* 2002;46:35–41.

Lozada-Nur F, Miranda C. Oral lichen planus: topical and systemic therapy. *Semin Cutan Med Surg* 1997;16:295–300.

Lundquist G, Forsgren H, Gajecki M, et al. Photochemotherapy of oral lichen planus: A controlled study. *Oral Surg Oral Med Oral Pathol Oral Radiol Endod* 1995;79:554–558.

Morrison L, Kratochvil FJ, Gorman A. An open trial of topical tacrolimus for erosive oral lichen planus. *J Am Acad Dermatol* 2002;47:617–620.

Scully C, Beyli M, Ferreiro MC, et al. Update on oral lichen planus: Etiopathogenesis and management. *Crit Rev Oral Biol Med* 1998;9:86–122.

Scully C, Eisen D, Carrozzo M. Management of oral lichen planus. *Am J Clin Dermatol* 2000;1:287–306.

Linear IgA Disease

■ Definition

Linear IgA disease is a rare, chronic, vesiculobullous mucocutaneous disorder characterized by a linear homogeneous deposition of IgA antibodies along the basement zone membrane.

■ Etiology

It is an autoimmune disease. The target antigens in linear IgA disease are multiple. The major antigen seems to be BP180, but others such as BP290, LAD_1, LAD_{285}, and collagen VII may also be target antigens.

■ Main Clinical Features

The oral mucosa is affected in about 20–25% of the cases and usually follow skin involvement. The oral lesions are indistinguishable from those seen in cicatricial pemphigoid.

Oral Mucosa

Localized or widespread bullae that rupture leaving painful erosions on the oral mucosa. Gingival involvement may be either in the form of *desquamative gingivitis* or as localized bullae and erosion

Other Mucosae

Rarely conjunctival, nasal, and laryngeal mucosae may be involved. Skin lesions are accompanied by pruritus and present as vesicles distributed in a symmetrical and cluster pattern. The vesicles rupture leaving erosions covered by crusts

Skin

The arms, buttocks, perioral skin, and genitalia are most frequently affected. Recurrence is common

■ Diagnosis

The clinical diagnosis should be confirmed by histopathologic examination and direct and indirect immunofluorescence tests.

■ Differential Diagnosis

- Cicatricial pemphigoid
- Bullous pemphigoid
- Epidermolysis bullosa acquisita
- Pemphigoid gestationis
- Dermatitis herpetiformis
- Pemphigus
- Chronic ulcerative stomatitis
- Bullous erythema multiforme

■ Treatment

Basic Guidelines

- The management of linear IgA disease consists of systemic or topical treatment depending on the severity of the disease and the organs involved.
- Patients with oral lesions should avoid mechanical injuries from rough foods, toothbrushes, broken teeth etc. Dentists must use dental instruments gently.
- Maintenance of excellent oral hygiene is necessary.

Suggested Therapies

Systemic Treatment

Dapsone

Dapsone is the treatment of choice for linear IgA disease. The usual, average dose to control the disease is 100 mg/day and then the dose is tapered every 3–6 weeks. Hemolytic anemia is the most severe side effect of dapsone. A blood count should be done every 2 weeks for the first 2 months of treatment and later every 1–2 months.

Sulfonamides

Sulfonamides, sulfapyridine 0.5–2 g/day, or sulfamethoxypyridazine 0.5–1.5 g/day may be used either alone or in combination with dapsone. The dose should be tapered every 3–6 weeks after control of the disease. Erythema multiforme, toxic epidermal necrolysis, agranulocytosis, and neutropenia are the more severe side effects of sulfonamide treatment.

Oral Corticosteroids

Oral corticosteroids, prednisone or prednisolone 20–80 mg/day, usually control the disease either alone or in combination with dapsone or sulfonamides. The dose of corticosteroids is slowly tapered every 2–3 weeks following adequate control of the disease.

Topical Treatment

Topical therapy with corticosteroids in an oral adhesive base (0.1% triamcinolone acetonide) or 0.5% fluocinonide gel or 0.05% clobetasol propionate gel, should be used to control oral lesions. The paste or gel is applied to the lesions two to three times daily for 2–6 weeks or longer. This type of treatment is particularly useful to control desquamative gingivitis. Intralesional injections of triamcinolone acetonide or betamethasone dipropionate and sodium phosphate are effective for localized oral lesions.

Alternative Therapies

Colchicine 0.1–1.5 mg/day, erythromycin 2 g/day, tetracycline 2 g/day and nicotinamide 1–2 g/day may be used as alternative treatments. High doses of intravenous immunoglobulin may also be used as adjunctive therapy for resistant cases. Cyclosporine is effective in the treatment of linear IgA disease.

References

Benbnisty KM, Bowman PH, Davis LS. Localized linear IgA disease responding to colchicine. *Int J Dermatol* 2002; 41:56–58.

Chorzelski TP, Jablonska S, Maciejowska E. Linear IgA bullous dermatosis of adults. *Clin Dermatol* 1992;9:383–392.

Cooper SM, Powell J, Wojnarowska F. Linear IgA disease: Successful treatment with erythromycin. *Clin Exp Dermatol* 2002;27:677–679.

Jolles S. A review of high-dose intravenous immunoglobulin in the treatment of the autoimmune blistering disorders. *Clin Exp Dermatol* 2001;26:127–131.

Wojnarowska F. What's new in linear IgA disease? *J Eur Acad Dermatol Venereol* 2000;14:441–443.

Wojnarowska F, Kirtschig G, Khumalo N. Treatment of subepidermal immunobullous diseases. *Clin Dermatol* 2001;19:768–777.

Young HS, Coulson IH. Linear IgA disease: Successful treatment with cyclosporin. *Br J Dermatol* 2000;143:204–205.

Ludwig Angina

▦ Definition

Ludwig angina is an acute, life-threatening infection of the sublingual and submandibular spaces and the floor of the mouth usually of odontogenic origin.

▦ Etiology

The causative organisms are staphylococci, streptococci, and anaerobic microorganisms.

▦ Main Clinical Features

- Erythema and edema of the floor of the mouth and the upper part of the neck under the chin
- Pain, sore throat, dysphagia, and drooling are common
- Tongue may be displaced upward and backward by the spreading infection. This, in association with spread of infection to the lateral pharyngeal spaces, may lead to occlusion of the airway
- Fever, chills, and malaise are common constitutional symptoms

▦ Diagnosis

The clinical diagnosis should be confirmed by a Gram smear and culture.

▦ Differential Diagnosis

- Suppurative sialadenitis
- Tuberculosis
- Mikulicz syndrome
- Sjögren syndrome
- Sarcoidosis
- HIV infection
- Salivary gland tumors
- Post-radiation cellulitis

▦ Treatment

Basic Guidelines

- Patients should be hospitalized.
- Intravenous antibiotics are necessary.
- Maintenance of the airway is important.
- External surgical drainage may also be required.

Suggested Therapies

- Intravenous penicillin G 6–12 megaunits every 6 hours and metronidazole 500 mg every 6 hours for 7–12 days is the regimen of choice.
- Parenteral cefotaxime 1–2 g every 6–12 hours plus metronidazole is an alternative regimen.
- Clindamycin or gentamicin are alternative choices.
- If airway patency is threatened tracheostomy is mandatory.
- Surgical drainage is occasionally necessary.

References

Barakate MS, Jensen MJ, Hemli JM, Graham AR. Ludwig's angina: report of a case and review of management issues. *Ann Otol Rhinol Laryngol* 2001;110:453–456.
Fritsch DE, Klein DG. Ludwig's angina. *Am J Infect Control* 1992;21:39–46.
Hutchinson IL, James DR. New treatment for Ludwig's angina. *Br J Oral Maxillofac Surg* 1989;27:83–84.
Parhiscar A, Har-El G. Deep neck abscess: A retrospective review of 210 cases. *Ann Otol Rhinol Laryngol* 2001;110: 1051–1054.

Lupus Erythematosus

▣ Definition

Lupus erythematosus is a chronic inflammatory autoimmune disease with a variable spectrum of clinical types in which mucocutaneous lesions may occur with or without systemic manifestations.

▣ Etiology

Lupus erythematosus is an autoimmune disease. Genetic, immunologic, infectious, drugs, and other factors may be involved in the pathogenesis.

▣ Main Clinical Features

There are two main types—discoid (cutaneous) and systemic (with multiple organ system involvement)—with intermediate subtypes. The oral mucosa is affected in both types: 15–20% of the discoid and 30–45% of the systemic cases develop oral lesions. Rarely, the oral lesions are the first sign of the disease.

Oral Lesions

- Atrophic red plaques surrounded by irradiating whitish striae, painful erosions or ulcers
- Petechiae, hemorrhages, edema, xerostomia
- White plaques and atrophic areas may be present

Other Mucosal Lesions

- Conjunctival, nasal, and genital mucosa may be involved

Skin Lesions

- Violaceous papules and patches, scaling and follicular hyperkeratosis, atrophy, telangiectasia, and scarring
- Characteristic "butterfly" pattern on the face
- Bullae formation may also be present.

Systemic Manifestations

- Fever, fatigue, weight loss, lymphadenopathy and debilitation
- Cardiovascular and gastrointestinal systems, lungs, kidneys, joints
- Central nervous system manifestations

▣ Diagnosis

The clinical diagnosis should be confirmed by histopathologic examination, direct immunofluorescence, serologic tests, and hematologic examination.

▣ Differential Diagnosis

- Lichen planus
- Chronic ulcerative stomatitis
- Cicatricial pemphigoid
- Bullous pemphigoid
- Linear IgA disease
- Dermatomyositis
- Graft-versus-host disease
- Drug-induced oral lesions
- Erythema multiforme
- Leukoplakia
- Erythroplakia

▣ Treatment

Basic Guidelines

- The treatment of lupus erythematosus should be undertaken by a specialist (dermatologist, rheumatologist, internist).
- The oral lesions should be managed by a specialist in oral medicine in collaboration with the other physicians involved in the treatment of lupus erythematosus.
- Maintenance of excellent oral hygiene is essential.
- Oral lesions may be treated systemically or locally depending on the severity and the type of lesions.
- Patients with skin lesions should avoid exposure to the sun.

Suggested Therapies

Systemic Treatment

Corticosteroids, immunosuppressants (azathioprine, cyclophosphamide, methotrexate, cyclosporine, mycophenolate mofetil), nonsteroidal anti-inflammatory drugs, and antimalarials have been used in the systemic treatment of lupus erythematosus. Thalidomide, dapsone, and retinoids may also be helpful in some cases.

Topical Treatment

Topical steroids (0.1% triamcinolone acetonide or 0.05% clobetasol) in an adhesive base (Orabase) should be applied on the oral lesions, two or three times a day for 3–6 weeks depending on the response. Intralesional injection of corticosteroids is also helpful, in particular for erosive lesions. Topical tacrolimus may also be used.

Oral lesions that do not respond to the above treatment may require administration of systemic corticosteroids (prednisone or prednisolone 20–30 mg/day) for 2–6 weeks if necessary. Hyperkeratotic oral lesions should be treated surgically.

References

Amato L, Coronella G, Berti S, et al. Subacute cutaneous lupus erythematosus in childhood. *Pediatr Dermatol* 2003;20:31–34.

Fivenson DP. Nonsteroidal treatment of autoimmune skin diseases. *Dermatol Clin* 1997;15:695–705.

Gescuk BD, Davis JC Jr. Novel therapeutic agents for systemic lupus erythematosus. *Curr Opin Rheumatol* 2002; 14:515–521.

Hanjani NM, Nousari CH. Mycophenolate mofetil for the treatment of cutaneous lupus erythematosus with smoldering systemic involvement. *Arch Dermatol* 2002; 138:1616–1618.

Housman TS, Jorizzo JL, McCarty MA, et al. Low-dose thalidomide therapy for refractory cutaneous lesions of lupus erythematosus. *Arch Dermatol* 2003;139:50–54.

Ioannou Y, Isenberg DA. Current concepts for the management of systemic lupus erythematosus in adults: a therapeutic challenge. *Postgrad Med J* 2002;78:599–606.

Patel P, Werth V. Cutaneous lupus erythematosus: A review. *Dermatol Clin* 2002;20:373–385.

Walker SL, Kirby B, Chalmers RJ. The effect of topical tacrolimus on severe recalcitrant chronic discoid lupus erythematosus. *Br J Dermatol* 2002;147:405–406.

Malignant Melanoma

▪ Definition

Malignant melanoma is a malignant neoplasm of the melanocytes.

▪ Etiology

The etiology is unknown. However, several risk factors, both genetic and environmental, have been implicated.

▪ Classification

On the basis of clinical and histopathological criteria malignant melanoma has been classified into four major types: a) superficial spreading melanoma, b) nodular melanoma, c) lentigo maligna melanoma, and d) acral lentiginous melanoma.

▪ Main Clinical Features

The incidence of malignant melanoma of the skin has dramatically increased over the past two decades and accounts for 15–30 per 100 000 individuals per year. Primary oral malignant melanoma is rare representing 0.5–1.5% of all malignant melanomas. The first three types of the neoplasm may develop in the oral mucosa.

- *Superficial spreading melanoma*: Circumscribed flat or slightly elevated brown or black plaque with irregular margins that spreads peripherally
- *Nodular melanoma*: Elevated black or reddish-brown nodule that grows quickly, hemorrhages easily, and may be ulcerated
- *Lentigo maligna melanoma*: Melanotic plaque or nodule that develops on a preexisting lentigo maligna lesion
- The palate, upper gingiva, and the alveolar mucosa are the most commonly affected areas

▪ Diagnosis

The clinical diagnosis should be confirmed by an excision biopsy and histopathologic examination.

▪ Differential Diagnosis

- Lentigo maligna
- Lentigo
- Freckles
- Pigmented nevi
- Amalgam tattoo
- Smoking-associated melanosis
- Melanoacanthoma
- Pyogenic granuloma
- Peripheral giant cell granuloma
- Kaposi sarcoma

▪ Treatment

Basic Guidelines

- Before deciding the treatment, the type of melanoma, depth and level of invasion, presence/absence of ulceration, and removal of lymph node metastases should be considered.
- Before treatment the tumor should be assessed according to the TNM classification proposed by the American Joint Committee on Cancer.
- The management of malignant melanoma includes prevention, early diagnosis, treatment and follow-up.
- Adjuvant therapies are occasionally initiated following by surgery.

Suggested Therapies

- Radical surgical excision is the mainstay of treatment. Regional lymph node dissection is undertaken in cases of positive sentinel lymph node biopsy and when palpable lymph nodes exist.
- Adjuvant therapy after surgical excision includes chemotherapy in combination with immunotherapy or hormonal therapy.
- Radiotherapy may provide effective palliation in advanced malignant melanoma.

References

Balch C, Buzaid AC, Atkins MB, et al. New American Joint Committee on Cancer Staging System for Cutaneous Melanoma. *Cancer* 2000;88:1484–1491.

Kirkwood JM. Adjuvant interferon in the treatment of melanoma. *Br J Cancer* 2000;82:1755–1756.

Kirkwood JM. Interferon (IFN) is the standard therapy of high-risk resectable cutaneous melanoma. *Melanoma Res* 2001;11(suppl 1):7.

Legha SS. Treatment of advanced melanoma with cytotoxic drugs. *Melanoma Res* 2001;11(suppl 1):13.

Medina JE, Ferlito A, Pellitteri PK, et al. Current management of mucosal melanoma of the head and neck. *J Surg Oncol* 2003;83:116–122.

Patel SG, Prasad ML, Escrig M, et al. Primary malignant melanoma of the head and neck. *Head Neck* 2002;24:247–257.

Sharpless SM, Das Cupta TK. Surgery for metastatic melanoma. *Semin Surg Oncol* 1998;14:311–318.

Median Lip Fissure

Definition

Median lip fissure is a relatively rare chronic inflammatory disorder of the midline of the lips.

Etiology

The exact cause is unknown. However, mechanical irritation, maceration, cold, sun exposure, windy and dry weather and atopy have been implicated as predisposing factors and probably a hereditary predisposition.

Main Clinical Features

- Deep, inflammatory, persistent and painful vertical fissure in the middle of the lip
- The lesion is usually infected by bacteria and *Candida albicans*
- Discomfort and spontaneous bleeding are common

Diagnosis

The diagnosis is exclusively based on the clinical features.

Treatment

Basic Guidelines

- Elimination of any possible predisposing factor.
- Avoid any mechanical pressure by foods and smiling during therapy.
- Recurrence is common.

Suggested Therapies

- Mild- or high-potency corticosteroid creams or ointments for about 2–4 weeks may be helpful. If a secondary infection is present, an ointment with antibiotics and antimycotics should be added.
- In severe, persistent cases resistant to corticosteroid therapy, surgical excision is the treatment of choice usually with good results.

References

Axel T, Skoglund A. Chronic lip fissures. *Int J Oral Surg* 1981;10:354–358.

Rosenquist BE. Median lip fissure: Etiology and suggested treatment. *Oral Surg Oral Med Oral Pathol* 1991;72:10–14.

Rosenquist BE. Median lip fissure. *J Craniofac Surg* 1995;6: 390–391.

Median Rhomboid Glossitis

Definition

Median rhomboid glossitis is a relatively rare disorder that characteristically appears in the midline of the posterior dorsum of the tongue.

Etiology

The defect is developmental in origin. However, recently it has been proposed that *Candida albicans* infection may play a role.

Main Clinical Features

- Well-demarcated, erythematous red plaque that is devoid of normal filiform papillae
- The lesion may be a uniform and smooth or a multinodular red plaque
- It is usually asymptomatic. However, when *Candida albicans* infection occurs subjecting symptoms such as a burning sensation and mild soreness may be present

Diagnosis

The diagnosis is based on the clinical features. Smear examination and culture for *Candida* may be done.

Differential Diagnosis

- Erythematous candidiasis
- Hemangioma
- Lymphangioma
- Geographic tongue
- Non-Hodgkin lymphoma
- Thyroglossal duct cyst

Treatment

- Median rhomboid glossitis is a benign disorder usually requiring no treatment. The patients should be reassured.
- In cases of *C. albicans* infection with subjective symptoms topical use of nystatin suspension or clotrimazole gel or even oral itraconazole 100 mg/day for 1–2 weeks may improve the symptoms.

References

Laskaris G. *Color Atlas of Oral Diseases*, 3rd edition. Thieme Verlag: Stuttgart, 2003.

Walsh LJ, Cleveland DB, Cumming CG. Quantitative evaluation of Langerhans cells in median rhomboid glossitis. *J Oral Pathol Med* 1992;21:28–33.

Van der Waal N. *Candida albicans* in median rhomboid glossitis: A post-mortem study. *Int J Oral Maxillofac Surg* 1986;15:322–325.

Melkersson–Rosenthal Syndrome

▓ Definition

Melkersson–Rosenthal syndrome, is a rare non-caseating granulomatous disease.

▓ Etiology

The etiology is unknown.

▓ Main Clinical Features

- Recurrent facial swelling
- Red, edematous swellings on the gingiva, buccal mucosa, tongue, and palate
- Labial swelling
- Recurrent unilateral facial palsy
- Fissured tongue
- Oral mucosal erosions
- Alteration of taste (rare)
- Hyposalivation (rare)

▓ Diagnosis

Biopsy and histopathologic examination may confirm the clinical diagnosis.

▓ Differential Diagnosis

- Peripheral facial nerve paralysis
- Angioedema
- Cheilitis granulomatosa
- Cheilitis glandularis
- Sarcoidosis
- Heerfordt syndrome
- Crohn disease
- Orofacial granulomatosis

▓ Treatment

Basic Guidelines

- Elimination of possible triggering factors such as dental foci of infection, other infections and foods.
- Persistent orofacial swelling of Melkersson–Rosenthal syndrome results in cosmetic and functional disabilities that requires surgical plastic reconstruction.
- Occasionally, the lesions may resolve spontaneously.
- In several cases the therapeutic regimens are unsuccessful.
- There is no specific treatment.

Suggested Therapies

- Systemic corticosteroids, e.g., prednisone 30–60 mg/day for 2–4 weeks and then tapering to and maintaining a dose of 10 mg/day for 2–4 months may successfully control the progression of the disease. However, recurrences are common.
- Antimalarials such as hydroxychloroquine or chloroquine and dapsone may also be used if corticosteroids fail to control the disease.
- Clofazimine, an antileprosy drug, has been used to treat Melkersson–Rosenthal syndrome because of its anti-inflammatory properties.
- Antibiotics such as minocycline 100–200 mg/day or metronidazole 250–500 mg three times daily for 1–3 months or more in combination with corticosteroids. Minocycline is used for its anti-inflammatory effects and because of its in-vitro ability to inhibit granuloma formation.
- Intralesional corticosteroids may used for local resistant swellings.
- Surgical plastic reconstruction has been used to improve permanent disfiguration of the lips.

References

Arbiser JL, Moschella SL. Clofazimine: A review of its medical used and mechanisms of action. *J Am Acad Dermatol* 1995;32:241–247.

Glickman LT, Gruss JS, Birt BD, Kohli-Dang N. The surgical management of Melkersson–Rosenthal syndrome. *Plast Reconstr Surg* 1992;89:815–821.

Roger RS III. Melkersson–Rosenthal syndrome and orofacial granulomatosis. *Dermatol Clin* 1996;14:371–379.

Stein SL, Mancini AJ. Melkersson–Rosenthal syndrome in childhood: Successful management with combination steroids and minocycline therapy. *J Am Acad Dermatol* 1999;41:746–748.

Sussman GL, Yang WH, Steinberg S. Melkersson–Rosenthal syndrome: clinical, pathologic and therapeutic considerations. *Ann Allergy* 1992;69:187–194.

Van der Waal RI, Schulten EA, van der Meij EH, et al. Cheilitis granulomatosa: Overview of 13 patients with long-term follow-up results of management. *Int J Dermatol* 2002;41:225–229.

Veller Fornasa C, Catalano P, Preserico A. Minocycline in granulomatous cheilitis: Experience with six cases. *Dermatology* 1992;185:220.

Zimmer WM, Roger RS III, Reeve CM, Sheridan PJ. Orofacial manifestations of Melkersson–Rosenthal syndrome: A study of 42 patients and review of 220 cases from the literature. *Oral Surg Oral Med Oral Pathol* 1992;74:610–619.

Metal Depositions

Definition

Metal depositions are uncommon pigmented oral lesions caused by significant heavy metal ingestion.

Etiology

Ingestion of lead, mercury, bismuth, silver, or arsenic that results in intoxication is the most common cause.

Main Clinical Features

Lead Poisoning

Blue-gray line on the marginal gingiva known as the gingival lead line, advanced periodontal disease, excessive salivation, metallic taste, and tremor of the tongue

Mercury Poisoning

Blue-gray gingiva, metallic taste, ulcerative stomatitis, salivary gland enlargement, premature exfoliation of teeth in children

Bismuth Poisoning

Blue-gray line on the marginal gingiva, similar to that seen in lead poisoning

Silver Poisoning

Slate-gray gingival margin line or diffuse discolorations of the same color apparent on the oral mucosa

Arsenic Poisoning

Excessive salivation, necrotizing ulcerative stomatitis and possibly, hyperkeratotic lesions mainly observed on the tongue

Diagnosis

The diagnosis is usually based on the medical history and the clinical features. Biopsy and histopathologic examination may occasionally be necessary to rule out other lesions.

Differential Diagnosis

- Amalgam tattoo
- Racial pigmentation
- Addison disease
- Von Recklinghausen disease
- Hemochromatosis
- Posttraumatic pigmentation
- Chronic pulmonary disease
- Pigmented nevi

Treatment

Basic Guidelines

- Removal of the causative agent.
- Supportive care.

Suggested Therapies

The use of chelating agents such as EDTA, BAL, DMSA or DMPS is the recommended course of action.

References

Aposhian HV, Maiorino RM, Rivera M, et al. Human studies with the chelating agents, DMPS and DMSA. *J Toxicol Clin Toxicol* 1992;30:505–528.

Chou CH, De Rosa CT. Case studies—arsenic. *Int J Hyg Environ Health* 2003;206:381–386.

Gordon JN, Taylor A, Bennett PN. Lead poisoning: Case studies. *Br Clin Pharmacol* 2002;53:451–458.

Keys DW, Nixon KC, Adkins KF. Oral manifestations of chronic lead-poisoning (plumbism): A case report. *N Z Dent J* 1973;69:205–208.

Mucormycosis

Definition

Mucormycosis is a rare, life-threatening opportunistic fungal infection characterized by vascular invasion and tissue necrosis.

Etiology

The causative organisms are fungi belonging to the family Mucoraceae, mainly *Rhizopus* and *Mucor* and, rarely, other species. Predisposing conditions are diabetes, hematologic malignancies, chronic renal failure, HIV disease, organ transplantation, and treatment with corticosteroids and cytotoxic drugs.

Classification

There are four clinical types of mucormycosis: a) rhinocerebral, b) pulmonary, c) gastrointestinal, and d) disseminated.

Main Clinical Features

The oral mucosa is affected in rhinocerebral mucormycosis. This type accounts for 40–70% of all reported cases.

Oral Manifestations

Palatal ulceration and necrosis are the most typical oral lesions. The sharply demarcated ulcer has a characteristic black necrotic eschar and bone is exposed. The surrounding mucosa is thickened

Other Signs and Symptoms

Low-grade fever, malaise, headache, sinus pain, bloody nasal discharge, periorbital and perinasal swelling and edema, eyelid ptosis, extraocular muscle paresis, and progressive lethargy are the most common signs and symptoms. Tissue necrosis in the nasal and paranasal sinuses may result in palatal perforation. Orbital and intracranial invasion is a common complication

Diagnosis

Biopsy and histopathologic examination of oral lesions is required for diagnosis. Computed tomography (CT) scan may be used to demonstrate bony lesions.

Differential Diagnosis

- Aspergillosis
- Paracoccidioidomycosis
- Cryptococcosis
- Malignant granuloma
- Wegener granulomatosis
- Non-Hodgkin lymphoma
- Squamous cell carcinoma
- Agranulocytosis
- *Pseudomonas aeruginosa* infection
- Gumma
- Necrotizing sialadenometaplasia

Treatment

Basic Guidelines

- The oral physician has an important role in the diagnosis of rhinocerebral mucormycosis.
- Early diagnosis and treatment are important to control the progress of the disease.
- Control and treatment of the underlying predisposing conditions are important for a successful outcome.
- Surgical and antifungal treatment are necessary.
- The treatment is primarily carried out by an internist specializing in infectious diseases.

Suggested Therapies

- Amphotericin B is the first-line drug for controlling the disease. A high dose of i.v. amphotericin B (1–1.5 mg/kg per day) must be started as soon as possible. This regimen should be administered only in a special hospital unit.
- Surgical removal of necrotic and nonperfused tissues as soon as possible is necessary.

References

Economopoulou P, Laskaris G, Ferekidis E, Kanelis N. Rhinocerebral mucormycosis with severe oral lesions: A case report. *J Oral Maxillofac Surg* 1995;53:215–219.

Hann IM, Prentice HG. Lipid-based amphotericin B: A review of the last 10 years of use. *Int J Antimicrob Agents* 2001;17:161–169.

Larsen K, Buchwald C, Ellefsen B, Francis D. Unexpected expansive paranasal sinus mucormycosis. *J Otorhinolaryngol Relat Spec* 2003;65:57–60.

Laskaris G. Oral manifestations of infectious diseases. *Dent Clin North Am* 1996;40:395–423.

Sellami-Boudawara T, Gouiaa N, Charfeddine I, et al. Facial mucormycosis: Observations from three cases. *Rev Stomatol Chir Maxillofac* 2002;103:369–372.

Mumps

▨ Definition

Mumps is an acute, self-limiting infectious disease that most frequently affects children 5–15 years of age and rarely older people.

▨ Etiology

The causative organism is a paramyxovirus.

▨ Main Clinical Features

The parotid gland and less often the submandibular and sublingual glands are predominantly affected. The incubation period is 14–21 days.

Salivary Gland Involvement

- Parotid tenderness with overlying facial edema
- Painful swelling of one or both of the parotids that last for about 7 days
- Orifice of the Stensen duct is usually red and swollen
- Variable swelling and tenderness of the submandibular and sublingual glands
- Occasionally, one gland subsides completely before the others become involved

Complications

- Orchitis
- Pancreatitis
- Meningitis
- Oophoritis

Constitutional Symptoms

- Variable fever and malaise
- Chills
- Headache

▨ Diagnosis

The diagnosis is confirmed by isolating the mumps virus from saliva or cerebrospinal fluid and serologic examination. The serum amylase may be elevated with relative lymphocytosis.

▨ Differential Diagnosis

- Acute suppurative parotitis
- Calculi in the parotid ducts
- Buccal cellulitis
- Angioedema
- Reaction to iodides
- Drug reaction
- Sjögren syndrome
- Mikulicz syndrome
- Sarcoidosis
- HIV infection
- Sialosis
- Salivary glands neoplasms
- Lymph node inflammation

▨ Treatment

Basic Guidelines

- Mumps vaccine is strongly recommended.
- The patient should be isolated for about 1 week and should stay in bed.
- The treatment is supportive. There is no specific antiviral therapy.
- The treatment of the complications must be undertaken by a specialist.

Suggested Therapies

- Analgesics and nonsteroidal anti-inflammatory agents may be used to control the parotid symptoms.
- Adequate hydration is necessary and soft food.
- Systemic corticosteroids should be avoided in the treatment of mumps.

References

Nardone A, Pebody RG, van den Hof S, et al. Sero-epidemiology of mumps in western Europe. *Epidemiol Infect* 2003;131:691–701.
Pugh RN, Akinosi B, Pooransingh S, et al. An outbreak of mumps in the metropolitan area of Walsall, UK. *Int J Infect Dis* 2002;6:283–287.

Necrotizing Sialadenometaplasia

◼ Definition

Necrotizing sialadenometaplasia is an acute, benign inflammatory lesion of the salivary glands.

◼ Etiology

The etiology is unknown, although it is believed that a vascular infarction leads to ischemic necrosis of the salivary tissues.

◼ Main Clinical Features

- Nodular swelling that leads to a painful crater-like ulcer with irregular and ragged borders.
- Diameter varies from 0.5 cm to 5 cm
- Sudden onset
- Posterior part of hard palate is the site of predilection followed by the lower lip, buccal mucosa, and occasionally the parotid gland
- Clinically the lesions mimic malignant neoplasms

◼ Diagnosis

The diagnosis should be confirmed by a biopsy and histopathologic examination.

◼ Differential Diagnosis

- Squamous cell carcinoma
- Mucoepidermoid carcinoma
- Other malignant types of adenocarcinomas
- Traumatic ulcer
- Malignant granuloma
- Non-Hodgkin lymphoma
- Syphilitic gumma
- Systemic mycoses

◼ Treatment

Basic Guidelines

- Biopsy is necessary to rule out malignancies.
- The lesion is usually self-limiting in about 4–10 weeks time.

Suggested Therapies

- Systemic oral corticosteroids in low doses, e. g., prednisone 10–20 mg/day for one week and 5–10 mg/day for one additional week dramatically improve the symptoms and help the lesions to heal quickly.
- Mouthwashes with oxygen releasing agents, e. g., carbamide peroxide may help to keep the surface of the ulcer clean and heal sooner, particularly if is used in conjunction with corticosteroids.
- Systemic antibiotics are only recommended if there is destruction of the underlying bone.

References

Brannon RB, Fowler CB, Hartman KS. Necrotizing sialometaplasia: A clinicopathological study of sixty-nine cases and review of the literature. *Oral Surg Oral Med Oral Pathol* 1991;72:317–325.

Koscielny S, Raabe G. Necrotizing sialometaplasia: A specific differential diagnosis of an ulcer of the hard palate. *Laryngorhinootologie* 2003;82:568–572.

Lombardi T, Samson J, Kuffer R. Subacute necrotizing sialadenitis: A form of necrotizing sialometaplasia? *Arch Otolaryngol Head Neck Surg* 2003;129:972–975.

Pulse Cl, Lebovics RS, Zegarelli DJ. Necrotizing sialometaplasia: Report of a case after lower lip mucocele excision. *J Oral Maxillofac Surg* 2002;58:1419–1421.

Necrotizing Ulcerative Gingivitis and Periodontitis

Definition

Necrotizing ulcerative gingivitis (NUG) is an acute or subacute gingival infection that usually affects young individuals. When the disease affects the deeper periodontal tissues with severe bone destruction the term necrotizing ulcerative periodontitis (NUP) is used.

Etiology

The cause is not fully understood. However, *Fusiform bacillus, Borrelia vincentii, Bacteroides gingivalis, Fusobacterium nucleatum, Prevotella intermedia*, and other anaerobic microorganisms are thought to play a role in the pathogenesis of the disease. Predisposing factors include emotional stress, poor oral hygiene, smoking, local trauma, HIV infections and immune defects.

Main Clinical Features

- Fiery red, swollen, and painful gingivae
- Necrosis and ulceration of the interdental papillae and the free margins of the gingivae
- Crater-like formation
- Spontaneous hemorrhage
- Intense salivation
- Halitosis
- Rapid periodontal bone destruction (only in necrotizing ulcerative periodontitis)
- Regional lymphadenopathy
- Low-grade fever and malaise
- Lesions may be localized or generalized
- Oral mucosa may be involved (necrotizing ulcerative stomatitis)

Diagnosis

The diagnosis is based exclusively on clinical criteria.

Differential Diagnosis

- Necrotizing ulcerative periodontitis/gingivitis

- Primary herpetic gingivostomatitis
- Streptococcal gingivostomatitis
- Scurvy
- Agranulocytosis
- Leukemia
- Langerhans cell histiocytosis
- Glycogen storage disease type 1b

Treatment

Basic Guidelines

- The treatment may be systemic or local depending on the severity of the disease.
- Local mechanical treatment should be avoided during the acute phase.
- Patients with NUG quickly respond to measures that reduce the microbial flora.
- Systemic antibiotics are necessary in the presence of systemic symptoms and signs, generalized and severe gingival destruction, and lack of response to local procedures.

Suggested Therapies

Systemic Treatment

Systemic antibiotics such as metronidazole 250–500 mg three times daily for 5–6 days is recommended for the intermediate and severe forms of NUG and NUP. This regimen immediately reduces the pain and discomfort and the gingival destruction. Oral penicillin and erythromycin may also be used as alternatives.

Topical Treatment

Local mouthwashes with 3% carbamide of peroxide (Unisept) or other oxygenating agents should be used alone or in association with metronidazole depending on disease severity. In mild cases local measures are enough to control the disease.

Plaque-control measures, scaling, root planing, and, occasionally, gingivectomy may be necessary. This mechanical regimen should follow the control of the acute phase of the disease with systemic or/and local agents.

References

Novak MJ. Necrotizing ulcerative periodontitis. *Ann Periodontol* 1999;4:74–77.

Robinson PG. Treatment of HIV-associated periodontal diseases. *Oral Dis* 1997;3(suppl 1):238–240.

Rowland RW. Necrotizing ulcerative gingivitis. *Ann Periodontol* 1999,4:65–73.

Wade Dn, Kerns DG. Acute necrotizing ulcerative gingivitis-periodontitis: A literature review. *Mil Med* 1998,163:337–342.

Nicotinic Stomatitis

▪ Definition

Nicotinic stomatitis is relatively common lesion of the palate.

▪ Etiology

Nicotinic stomatitis is thought to represent the thermal injury caused by the heat generated during smoking. The benign nature of nicotinic stomatitis lends support to the theory that the chemical carcinogens present in tobacco play a minor role in its etiology.

▪ Main Clinical Features

- Diffuse red lesion of the palate that soon becomes a white-gray keratotic patch punctured with red dots
- Often characterized by fissures, furrows and plaques all representing different extents of keratinization of the oral epithelium. The red spots represent the inflamed orifices of the salivary gland ducts
- No pain or discomfort is associated with the lesion which does not detach

▪ Diagnosis

The clinical appearance is characteristic and is usually adequate for diagnosis.

▪ Differential Diagnosis

- Friction keratosis
- Leukoplakia
- Squamous cell carcinoma
- Candidiasis
- Lichen planus
- White sponge nevus

▪ Treatment

Basic Guidelines

- Nicotinic stomatitis is usually reversible. The palate returns to normal 2–6 weeks after smoking cessation.
- Any white lesion persisting on the palatal mucosa after 1 month of smoking cessation should be biopsied as it probably represents a leukoplakia.
- Nicotinic stomatitis indicates that the patient is at risk for developing a precancerous or cancerous lesion in another location in the oral cavity.
- Intraoral screening should be done every 6 months.

Suggested Therapies

Smoking cessation.

References

Andersson G, Vala EK, Curvall M. The influence of cigarette consumption and smoking machine yields of tar and nicotine on the nicotine uptake and oral mucosal lesions in smokers. *J Oral Pathol Med* 1997;26:117–123.

Gavarsana S, Sussarla MD. Palatal mucosal changes among reverse smokers in an Indian village. *Japn J Cancer Res* 1989;80:209–211.

Gupta PC, Murti PR, Bhonsle RB. Effect of cessation of tobacco use on the incidence of oral mucosal lesions in a 10-yr follow-up study of 12 212 users. *Oral Dis* 1995;1:54–58.

Ramulu C, Ratnam GV, Kameswari VR. Regression of stomatitis nicotine in reverse smokers. *Indian J Med Res* 1973;61:1328–1334.

Reibel J. Tobacco and oral diseases. Update on the evidence, with recommendations. *Med Princ Pract* 2003;12 (suppl 1):22–32.

Noma

■ Definition

Noma or cancrum oris is a rare, rapidly progressive and severe destructive disease usually involving the oral tissues.

■ Etiology

Fusospirochetal microorganisms, *Staphylococcus aureus, Streptococcus* species and *Pseudomonas aeruginosa* are almost always present. Predisposing factors are severe protein malnutrition, diabetes mellitus, hematologic malignancies, HIV infection, poor oral hygiene, dehydration, and systemic infectious diseases, particularly measles.

■ Main Clinical Features

The disease predominantly affects children in sub-Saharan Africa and it is extremely rare in Europe and North America.

- In most cases the infection begins as acute necrotizing ulcerative gingivitis that quickly spreads to the neighboring oral tissues
- Gangrenous necrosis of the cheeks, lips, and the underlying bone, produce catastrophic lesions on the face
- Gangrenous ulcers are covered with black or whitish-brown fibrin and debris
- Salivation
- Halitosis
- Fever, malaise, pain
- Regional lymphadenopathy
- Death is common

■ Diagnosis

The diagnosis is usually based on clinical criteria. Smear microscopy and culture may be done.

■ Differential Diagnosis

- Malignant granuloma
- Burkitt lymphoma
- Leukemia
- Agranulocytosis
- Aplastic anemia
- Oral malignancies
- Syphilis
- Tuberculosis

■ Treatment

Basic Guidelines

- The treatment must begin as soon as possible.
- A nutritious diet, rich in proteins and vitamins, is necessary.
- Hydration and correction of electrolyte imbalances are important for treatment.
- Treatment of predisposing disease is necessary.
- If the patient survives, scarring may produce oral stenosis requiring plastic surgery to prevent starvation.
- Mortality is 10–20%.

Suggested Therapies

Systemic Treatment

Antibiotics such as high-dose i.v. penicillin (10–20 MIU daily) and metronidazole 2–3 g/day are the drugs of choice for the treatment of noma. If *Pseudomonas aeruginosa* infection is present, gentamicin or ciprofloxacin (Ciproxin) are also indicated.

Topical Treatment

Oxygenating agents should be used along with conservative debridement of necrotic tissues. Chlorhexidine gluconate (0.2%) oral solution may be also used.

Surgical reconstruction should follow after stabilization of tissue destruction or sometimes even in the acute phase.

References

Adekeye EO, Ord RA. Cancrum oris: Principles of management and reconstructive surgery. *J Maxillofac Surg* 1983;11:160–170.

Baratti-Mayer D, Pittet B, Montandon D, et al. Noma: an "infectious" disease of unknown aetiology. *Lancet Infect Dis* 2003;3:419–431.

Berthold P. Noma: A forgotten disease. *Dent Clin North Am* 2003;47:559–574.

Enwonwu CO, Falkler WA Jr, Idigbe EO, Savage KO. Noma (cancrum oris): Questions and answers. *Oral Dis* 1999;5:144–149.

Marck KW, de Bruijn HP. Surgical treatment of noma. *Oral Dis* 1999;5:167–171.

Non-Hodgkin Lymphomas

▊ Definition

Non-Hodgkin lymphomas are a complex group of lymphoid tissue malignancies. About 90% of non-Hodgkin lymphomas originate from the B-lymphocyte series and 10% from the T-lymphocytes.

▊ Etiology

The etiology remains unknown. However, genetic and environmental factors (viruses, radiation, drugs) may be involved in the pathogenesis.

▊ Main Clinical Features

Oral non-Hodgkin lymphomas account for less than 5% of all oral malignancies. Over 80% of the disease arises in the Waldeyer ring and the palate. In the oral soft tissues lymphomas usually develop as extranodal disease and may represent local disease, but more frequently they represent part of widespread disease (lymphoma).

- Oral lesions present as diffuse, persistent, soft or firm, usually asymptomatic swellings that may ulcerate
- Lesion may be normal in color or reddish
- Mild pain or discomfort and paresthesias are common symptoms
- The soft palate, the posterior gingiva, the base of the tongue, floor of the mouth, and the peritonsillar region are the most frequent oral sites

▊ Diagnosis

The clinical diagnosis should be confirmed by histopathologic and immunocytochemical examination. Bone marrow biopsy, radiographs, and CT scans are also necessary.

▊ Differential Diagnosis

- Dental abscess
- Periodontal disease
- Malignant granuloma
- Necrotizing sialadenometaplasia
- Wegener granulomatosis
- Salivary gland tumors
- Squamous cell carcinoma
- Eosinophilic ulcer
- Tuberculosis
- Systemic mycoses

▊ Treatment

Basic Guidelines

- The treatment of oral lesions is supportive.
- The systemic treatment must be carried out by a specialist.

Suggested Therapies

Low-Grade Lymphomas

In this highly heterogeneous group of malignancies, treatment strategy may include curative irradiation, oral therapy usually with chlorambucil with or without prednisone, i.v. combination chemotherapy including COP (cyclophosphamide, vincristine, prednisone), CHOP (cyclophosphamide, doxorubicin, vincristine, prednisone), FND (fludarabine, mitoxantrone, dexamethasone) or i.v. monoclonal antibodies (anti-CD20 [MabThera]). Anti-CD20 antibody may be given either in combination with the aforementioned regimens or as a single agent therapy. For localized low-grade lymphomas radiation therapy may be curative. When the disease spreads to the skin s.c. interferon alpha can be given.

High-Grade Lymphomas

High-grade lymphomas are also a heterogeneous group of diseases. So far the standard treatment for B-cell high-grade lymphomas is the combination of MabThera and CHOP, while CHOP is used for T-cell lymphomas. Several alternative combinations are also available, either for patients who have had a relapse or for those with very aggressive disease. In selected patients high-dose chemotherapy combined with autologous stem cell support may be considered.

References

Bessell EM, Burton A, Haynes AP, et al. A randomised multicentre trial of modified CHOP versus MCOP in patients aged 65 years and over with aggressive non-Hodgkin's lymphoma. *Ann Oncol* 2003;14:258–267.

Doussis-Anagnostopoulou I, Pangalis GA, Kittas C. Extranodal lymphomas: A review. *Haema* 2001;4:215–229.

Epstein JB, Epstein JD, Le ND, Gorsky M. Characteristics of oral and paraoral malignant lymphoma: A population-based review of 361 cases. *Oral Surg Oral Med Oral Pathol Oral Radiol Endod* 2001;92:519–525.

Forero A, Lobuglio AF. History of antibody therapy for non-Hodgkin's lymphoma. *Semin Oncol* 2003;30(suppl 17): 1–5.

Gustavsson A, Osterman B, Cavallin-Stahl E. A systematic overview of radiation therapy effects in non-Hodgkin's lymphoma. *Acta Oncol* 2003;42:605–619.

Hauke RJ, Armitage JO. A new approach to non-Hodgkin's lymphoma. *Intern Med* 2000;39:197–208.

Horning SJ. Future directions in radioimmunotherapy for B-cell lymphoma. *Semin Oncol* 2003;30(suppl 17):29–34.

Jordan RC, Speight PM. Extranodal non-Hodgkin's lymphoma of the oral cavity. *Curr Top Pathol* 1996;90:125–146.

Mounter PJ, Lennard AL. Management of non-Hodgkin's lymphomas. *Postgrad Med J* 1999;75:2–6.

Reiser M, Diehl V. Current treatment of follicular non-Hodgkin's lymphoma. *Eur J Cancer* 2002;38:1167–1172.

Richards A, Costelloe MA, Eveson JN, et al. Oral mucosal non-Hodgkin's lymphoma—a dangerous mimic. *Oral Oncol* 2000;36:556–558.

Saubeyran P, Debled M, Tchen N, et al. Follicular lymphomas: A review of treatment modalities. *Crit Rev Oncol Hematol* 2000;35:13–32.

Oral Malodor

Definition

Oral malodor or halitosis or bad breath is a foul odor detected on exhalation. It is a symptom and not a disease entity.

Etiology

Oral malodor is multifactorial. Oral microorganisms, particularly Gram-negative anaerobes on the teeth and tongue, in association with protein remnants in the mouth are central to the production of oral malodor. Volatile and odorous agents such as hydrogen sulfide, methyl mercaptans and other sulfur-containing amino acids are the causes of the malodor. In over 92–95% of the cases the mouth is the origin of halitosis. The nasal passages constitute the second most frequent source of bad breath followed by some systemic diseases.

Main Clinical Features

- Bad breath is usually the only symptom. Individuals appear to be unaware of their own breath which is obvious to others
- Bacteria in the dental plaque and in the center of the dorsum of the tongue are thought to be the main reservoirs for the malodor producing microorganisms
- The best standard of bad breath measurement is the human nose
- Signs and other symptoms may be present if there is an underlying local or systemic disease

Diagnosis

The diagnosis is usually based on clinical observation. However, gas chromatography and gas monitors have been used to measure bad breath.

Differential Diagnosis

The differential diagnosis includes several local and systemic diseases that may produce bad breath.

Treatment

Basic Guidelines

- Oral malodor is a common complaint which presents in a dental office.
- Before treatment the exact origin of bad breath must be determined.
- Collaboration between the oral clinician (stomatologist), the otorhinolaryngologist, and the internist is sometimes necessary. Treatment of renal and other systemic diseases producing malodor is a priority.
- If the patient has poor oral hygiene, periodontal disease, and dental caries, these conditions must be treated before any topical antimicrobial or systemic treatment.
- Regular brushing of the dorsum of the tongue with a tongue cleaner or with a toothbrush once or twice daily over a long period of time is thought to be an important step in decreasing the odorgenic bacterial load.
- Recurrence of malodor is common.

Suggested Therapies

In severe and chronic malodor, systemic metronidazole 500 mg every 12 hours for 8–12 days followed by oxygen-releasing mouthwashes twice daily for one month and then once daily for one more month is, in my experience, the best therapeutic regimen. The malodor usually disappears in a day or two and the local mouthwash stabilizes the good result.

Chlorhexidine gluconate 0.2% mouthwash two to three times daily for several weeks may temporarily improve the condition. However, the bitter taste and subsequent discoloration of teeth preclude long-term usage.

Mouthwashes with cetylpyridinium chloride, benzethonium chloride, zinc ions, phenolic oils, two-phase oil and water mouthrinses, and several other local approaches to treatment either alone or in combination have been proposed for the treatment of oral malodor.

References

Borden LC, Chaves ES, Bowman JP, et al. The effect of four mouthrinses on oral malodor. *Compend Contin Educ Dent* 2002;23:531–536.

Cicek Y, Orbak R, Tezel A, et al. Effect of tongue brushing on oral malodor in adolescents. *Pediatr Int* 2003;45:719–723.

Loesche WJ. Microbiology and treatment of halitosis. *Curr Infect Dis Rep* 2003;5:220–226.

Quirynen M. Management of oral malodour. *J Clin Periodontol* 2003;30(suppl 5):17–18.

Roldan S, Winkel EG, Herrera D, et al. The effects of a new mouthrinse containing chlorhexidine, cetylpyridium chloride and zinc lactate on the microflora of oral halitosis patients: a dual-centre, double-blind placebo-controlled study. *J Clin Periodontol* 2003;30:427–434.

Rosenberg M (Editor). Bad breath: research perspectives. *Ramot Publ Tel Aviv Univ* 1995.

Rosenberg M, Gelernter I, Barki M, Bar-Ness R. Day-long reduction of oral malodor by a two phase oil: Water mouthrinse as compared to chlorhexidine and placebo rinse. *J Periodontol* 1992;63:39–43.

Yeung S. Oral malodour and its clinical management. *Ann R Australas Coll Dent Surg* 2002;16:141–144.

Young A, Jonski G, Rolla G. Inhibition of orally produced volatile sulfur compounds by zinc, chlorhexidine or cetylpyridinium chloride effect of concentration. *Eur J Oral Sci* 2003;111:400–404.

Oral Soft-Tissue Abscess

■ Definition

Oral soft-tissue abscesses are relatively uncommon resulting from infections of nondental origin.

■ Etiology

Staphylococcus aureus, β-hemolytic *Streptococcus* and less frequently anaerobic microorganisms are the cause.

■ Main Clinical Features

- Ill-defined, usually painful, swelling
- Hard or semihard on palpation
- Occasionally asymptomatic
- The tongue and buccal mucosa are more frequently affected

■ Diagnosis

The diagnosis is usually based on clinical criteria. Smear stain and culture may be useful.

■ Differential Diagnosis

- Actinomycosis
- Tuberculosis
- Benign tumors
- Foreign bodies

■ Treatment

- Oral dicloxacillin 250–500 mg every 8 hours for 6–8 days or flucloxacillin 250–500 mg every 8 hours for 6–8 days is recommended.
- Oral cephalexin 250–500 mg every 8 hours for 4–8 days or other cephalosporins may be used with success.
- Macrolides such as oral erythromycin 250–500 mg every 8 hours or oral clarithromycin 250–500 mg every 12 hours for 4–6 days may be used as an alternative therapy.
- Metronidazole 250–500 mg every 8 hours may also be used either alone or in combination with one of the above antibiotics.
- Drainage is important for quick and safe treatment.

References

Carrasco DA, Tyring SK. Skin and soft tissues infections. In: Finch RG, Greenwood D, Norrby SR, Whitley RJ (editors). *Antibiotics and Chemotherapy*, 8th edition. Churchill Livingstone: London, 2003.

Kuriyama T, Karasawa T, Nakagawa K, et al. Antimicrobial susceptibility of major pathogens of orofacial odontogenic infections to 11 beta-lactam antibiotics. *Oral Microbiol Immunol* 2002;17:285–289.

Laskaris G. *Color Atlas of Oral Diseases*, 3rd edition. Thieme Verlag: Stuttgart, 2003.

Oral Staphylococcal Infection

▨ Definition

Oral soft-tissue staphylococcal infection is a rare acute infection.

▨ Etiology

Staphylococcus aureus, Staphylococcus epidermidis, and rarely other strains are responsible.

▨ Main Clinical Features

- Round or oval ulceration with raised borders covered by a whitish or brown-white necrotic exudate
- Fever
- Malaise
- Regional lymphadenopathy

▨ Diagnosis

The clinical diagnosis should be confirmed by smear microscopy and culture.

▨ Differential Diagnosis

- Traumatic ulcer
- Streptococcal infection
- *Klebsiella* infection
- Aphthous ulcer
- Necrotizing ulcerative stomatitis
- Syphilitic ulcer (chancre)
- Eosinophilic ulcer
- Cyclic neutropenia
- Myelodysplastic syndrome
- Wegener granulomatosis

▨ Treatment

Basic Guidelines

- Smear microscopy and culture is always necessary before treatment.
- Early diagnosis and treatment is important.
- Systemic antibiotics are indicated and should be supplemented by topical antiseptics.

Suggested Therapies

Systemic Treatment

- Penicillinase-resistant penicillins such as oral dicloxacillin 250–500 mg every 8 hours daily or flucloxacillin 250–500 mg every 8 hours daily for 4–6 days are recommended.
- Oral cephalexin 250–500 mg every 8 hours daily for about 4–6 days is also effective.
- Oral macrolides such as erythromycin tablets 250–500 mg four times daily, or clarithromycin 250–500 mg twice daily, or azithromycin 250–500 mg/day for 4–6 days may be used as an alternative regimen.

Topical Treatment

Chlorhexidine gluconate 0.2% may be used as mouthwash three to four times daily.

References

Laskaris G. *Color Atlas of Oral Diseases*, 3rd edition. Thieme Verlag: Stuttgart, 2003.
Storoe W, Haug RH, Lillich TT. The changing face of odontogenic infections. *J Maxillofac Surg* 2001;59:739–748.

Oral Submucous Fibrosis

Definition

Oral submucous fibrosis is a chronic collagen disorder affecting the submucosal oral tissues resulting in limited tongue mobility and mouth opening. It is a precancerous condition. The disorder is common in India and other Asian countries, but sporadic cases have been recorded elsewhere in the world.

Etiology

The exact etiology remains unknown. However, betel nut chewing, areca nut, chili, tobacco products, smokeless tobacco products (gutkha), and vitamin B deficiency have been considered as possible etiologic agents.

Main Clinical Features

- Intense burning sensation and vesicle formation followed by erosions, salivation, and hypermelanosis
- The oral mucosa becomes progressively smooth, atrophic, and inelastic, as in scleroderma. The tongue is smooth, the uvula is destroyed, and multiple fibrotic bands develop.
- Opening of the mouth, mastication, and swallowing may be restricted
- About 5–10% of patients with submucous fibrosis develop squamous cell carcinoma

Diagnosis

The diagnosis should be confirmed by a biopsy and histopathologic examination.

Differential Diagnosis

- Tobacco pouch keratosis
- Leukoplakia
- Scleroderma
- Porphyria
- Cicatricial pemphigoid
- Atrophic lichen planus

- Pernicious anemia
- Plummer–Vinson syndrome

Treatment

Basic Guidelines

- A biopsy is necessary before treatment to determine the presence of epithelial dysplasia or to rule out carcinoma.
- The patients should be closely followed-up because of the high risk of malignant transformation.
- Avoidance of possible etiologic factors should be emphasized to the patients.
- The treatment is symptomatic and not curative.

Suggested Therapies

- Systemic oral corticosteroids, e.g., prednisone 20–30 mg/day for 2–4 weeks and then tapering the dose and discontinuing in about 1–2 months may help in the early stages of the disease.
- Topical corticosteroids, intralesional injection or ointments have also been used in localized lesions with temporary effect.
- Recently, intralesional injection of interferon gamma has been shown to have significant therapeutic effect on oral submucous fibrosis. The effect of interferon gamma on collagen synthesis appears to be the key to the treatment of these patients.
- Several surgical procedures have been suggested to improve mouth opening in severe cases and to prevent malignant transformation.
- Recently it has been proposed that oral administration of immunized cows' milk may improve the symptoms and signs in patients with oral submucous fibrosis.

References

Celik N, Wei FC, Chang YM, et al. Squamous cell carcinoma of the oral mucosa after release of submucous fibrosis and bilateral small radial forearm flap reconstruction. *Plast Reconstr Surg* 2002;110:34–38.

Haque MF, Meghji S, Nazir R, Harris M. Interferon gamma (IFN-gamma) may reverse oral submucous fibrosis. *J Oral Pathol Med* 2001;30:12–21.

Laskaris G, Bovopoulou O, Nicolis G. Oral submucous fibrosis in a Greek female. *Br J Oral Surg* 1981;19:197–201.

Tai YS, Liu BY, Wang JT, et al. Oral administration of milk from cows immunized with human intestinal bacteria leads to significant improvements of symptoms and signs in patients with oral submucous fibrosis. *J Oral Pathol Med* 2001;30: 618–625.

Tsai CH, Chou MY, Chang YC. The up-regulation of cyclooxygenase-2 expression in human buccal mucosal fibroblasts by arecoline: A possible role in the pathogenesis of oral submucous fibrosis. *J Oral Pathol Med* 2003;32: 146–153.

Wei FC, Chang YM, Kildal M, et al. Bilateral small radial forearm flaps for the reconstruciton of buccal mucosa after surgical release of submucous fibrosis: A new reliable approach. *Plast Reconstr Surg* 2001;107:1679–1683.

Orofacial Granulomatosis

Definition

Orofacial granulomatosis is a rare, heterogeneous, noninfectious disorder characterized by chronic swelling of the facial and oral tissues due to noncaseating granulomatous formation in patients with no other systemic granulomatous disease.

Etiology

The etiology of most cases is unknown. In several cases orofacial granulomatosis is a manifestation of Crohn disease, sarcoidosis, or Melkersson–Rosenthal syndrome.

Main Clinical Features

In several cases the diagnosis is made by exclusion of other systemic granulomatous diseases involving the orofacial region. However, occasionally orofacial involvement may be the initial presentation of these diseases.

- Lip swelling and enlargement
- Diffuse facial swelling
- Gingival swelling and erythema
- Buccal and palatal swelling
- Tongue swelling
- Oral ulceration
- Mucosal tags
- Burning and itching are common

Diagnosis

The clinical diagnosis should be confirmed by a biopsy and histopathologic examination.

Differential Diagnosis

- Crohn disease
- Sarcoidosis
- Melkersson–Rosenthal syndrome
- Tuberculosis
- Angioedema
- Cheilitis glandularis

Treatment

Basic Guidelines

- Other systemic granulomatous diseases should be excluded prior to treatment.
- In most patients orofacial granulomatosis is relatively asymptomatic.
- Management of orofacial granulomatosis depends on accurate diagnosis of the condition and recognition of any precipitating factors.
- If there is an underlying systemic condition, appropriate treatment for that condition may result in concomitant improvement of orofacial lesions.

Suggested Therapies

- Systemic corticosteroids, minocycline and other tetracyclines, dapsone, clofazimine, thalidomide, and hydroxychloroquine may be used in the treatment of orofacial granulomatosis.
- Intralesional corticosteroids may also be used in selected localized cases.
- Plastic surgery may be required in severe persistent cases.
- (For details see treatment of Melkersson–Rosenthal syndrome, cheilitis granulomatosa, Crohn disease, and sarcoidosis.)

References

Bogenrieder T, Rogler G, Vogt T, et al. Orofacial granulomatosis as the initial presentation of Crohn disease in an adolescent. *Dermatology* 2003;206:273–278.

Hegarty A, Hodgson T, Porter S. Thalidomide for the treatment of recalcitrant oral Crohn's disease and orofacial granulomatosis. *Oral Surg Oral Med Oral Pathol Oral Radiol Endod* 2003;95:576–585.

Rees TD. Orofacial granulomatosis and related conditions. *Periodontol 2000* 1999;21:145–157.

Sciubba JJ, Said-Al-Naief N. Orofacial granulomatosis: presentation, pathology and management of 13 cases. *J Oral Pathol Med* 2003;32:576–585.

Paracoccidioidomycosis

▓ Definition

Paracoccidioidomycosis, formerly known as South American blastomycosis, is a chronic systemic fungus disease that occur exclusively in Central and South America or in individuals who have lived in these areas.

▓ Etiology

The causative organism is *Paracoccidioides brasiliensis.*

▓ Main Clinical Features

The disease primarily infects the lungs. The skin, mucosae, lymph nodes, adrenal glands, and other organs may be affected.

Oral Lesions

The oral lesions present as chronic irregular ulcers with a granular surface. Palatal perforation may occur in severe cases. The palate, tongue, and gingiva are frequently involved.

Other Manifestations

The nose, larynx, and oropharynx, are usually the first sites of involvement and present ulcerations. Ulcerated papules on the skin and lymph node enlargement are also common. Cough, dyspnea, fever, weight loss, and gastrointestinal symptoms may occur.

▓ Diagnosis

Biopsy and histopathologic examination, smear and cultures, and serology may be useful for diagnosis.

▓ Differential Diagnosis

- Coccidioidomycosis
- Histoplasmosis
- Other systemic mycoses
- Tuberculosis
- Syphilis
- Sarcoidosis
- Wegener granulomatosis
- Leishmaniasis
- Malignant granuloma
- Squamous cell carcinoma
- Malignant salivary glands tumor
- Sialadenometaplasia

▓ Treatment

Basic Guidelines

- The oral lesions are usually part of systemic disease.
- The treatment of oral lesions should always be undertaken in collaboration with the specialist physician (infectious diseases).
- Long-term treatment is necessary.

Suggested Therapies

- Itraconazole 100–200 mg/day for 3–6 months is the treatment of choice for paracoccidioidomycosis. The clinical response is usually very good within 1 month but 3–6 months of treatment is necessary to avoid recurrences. The efficacy of itraconazole is comparable with ketoconazole, but it is better tolerated.
- Ketoconazole 200–400 mg/day for 3–6 months is also effective and the drug of second choice for the treatment of paracoccidioidomycosis.
- Amphotericin B is also effective. However, this drug should be used only in severe cases and those resistant to other drugs because of the severity of the side effects.

Future Therapies

Terbinafine, an allylamine, is a new option as drug therapy for paracoccidioidomycosis.

References

Achenbach R, Negroni R, Khaski S, et al. Paracoccidioidomycosis: Unusual clinical presentation and utility of computerized tomography scanning for diagnosis. *Int J Dermatol* 2002;41:881–882.

Almeida OP, Jorge J, Scully C. Paracoccidioidomycosis of the mouth: An emerging deep mycosis. *Crit Rev Oral Biol Med* 2003;14:268–274.

Bicalho RN, Santo MF, de Aguiar MC, Santos VR. Oral paracoccidioidomycosis: A retrospective study of 62 Brasilian patients. *Oral Dis* 2001;7:56–60.

Brummer E, Castaneda E, Restrepo A. Paracoccidioidomycosis: an update. *Clin Microbiol Rev* 1993;6:89–95.

Dismukes WE. Introduction to antifungal drugs. *Clin Infect Dis* 2000;30:653–657.

Hahn RC, Fontes CJ, Batista RD, Hamdan JS. In vitro comparison of activities of terbinafine and itraconazole against *Paracoccidioides brasiliensis*. *J Clin Microbiol* 2002;40:2828–2831.

Pellagra

■ Definition

Pellagra is the classic manifestation of vitamin B_3 or niacin deficiency.

■ Etiology

Deficiency of vitamin B_3 (niacin or nicotinic acid) due to alcoholism, nutrient–drug interactions, gastrointestinal diseases, anorexia nervosa, and genetic errors of metabolism leads to pellagra.

■ Main Clinical Features

The oral mucosa is commonly affected. The classic triad of pellagra is dermatitis, diarrhea, and dementia.

Oral Manifestations

- Edema, redness, and intense burning sensation
- Smooth, depapillated tongue with painful ulcers
- Gingivitis, dry and fissured lips, angular cheilitis, dysphagia
- Symmetric erythema of sun-exposed skin with scaling

Other Manifestations

- Skin desquamation and crusting, bulla formation, and hyperpigmentation are common
- Diarrhea, abdominal pain, and achlorhydria may occur
- Dementia: the patients are irritable, anxious, depressed, and apathetic
- If left untreated the disease is lethal

■ Diagnosis

The diagnosis is usually based on the clinical features. In early cases the diagnosis may be confirmed by measuring niacin metabolites in the urine.

■ Differential Diagnosis

- Ariboflavinosis
- Vitamin C deficiency
- Nutritional deficiencies
- Porphyrias
- Drug-induced stomatitis
- Erythema multiforme

■ Treatment

Basic Guidelines

- Foods containing high quantities of vitamin B_3 (red meat, liver, salmon) should be recommended.
- Stop intake of alcoholic drinks.
- A high-protein diet is also helpful.

Suggested Therapies

- Oral niacin 100–300 mg/day for about 2–3 weeks is the treatment of choice with a quick and excellent response.
- High level of oral hygiene is also recommended for improvement of oral lesions.

References

Hegyi J, Schwartz RA, Hegyi V. Pellagra: Dermatitis, dementia, and diarrhea. *Int J Dermatol* 2004;43:1–5.

Karthikeyan K, Thappa DM. Pellagra and skin. *Int J Dermatol* 2002;41:476–481.

Lyon VB, Fairley JA. Anticonvulsant-induced pellagra. *J Am Acad Dermatol* 2002;46:597–599.

Prousky JE. Pellagra may be a rare secondary complication of anorexia nervosa: a systematic review of the literature. *Altern Med Rev* 2003;8:180–185.

Pemphigoid Gestationis

▧ Definition

Pemphigoid gestationis or herpes gestationis is a rare, usually self-limiting, acute autoimmune subepidermal blistering disease occurring in the second or third trimester of pregnancy or in the early postpartum period.

▧ Etiology

Pemphigoid gestationis is an autoimmune disease. The autoimmune response in pemphigoid gestationis is mainly directed to a 180 kD hemidesmosomal antigen (BP180) or basal keratinocytes.

▧ Main Clinical Features

Pemphigoid gestationis usually affects the skin and, rarely, the mucous membranes (20%). A predominantly oral involvement is uncommon.

Oral Mucosa

- Multiple bullae that rupture leaving painful erosions
- The buccal mucosa, palate, lips, tongue, and rarely the gingiva are most frequently affected

Other Mucosae

- Conjunctival, vaginal, anal
- Inflammation, bullae, and erosions are the main lesions

Skin

- Pruritic papulovesicular eruptions, frequently generalized
- The lesions usually begin on the abdomen with a predilection for the periumbilical region, palms, and soles of the feet

▧ Diagnosis

The clinical diagnosis should be confirmed by histopathologic examination and direct and indirect immunofluorescence tests.

▧ Differential Diagnosis

- Cicatricial pemphigoid
- Bullous pemphigoid
- Linear IgA disease
- Epidermolysis bullosa acquisita
- Pemphigus
- Dermatitis herpetiformis
- Erythema multiforme
- Bullous systemic lupus erythematosus
- Drug eruptions

▧ Treatment

Basic Guidelines

- Systemic treatment is usually necessary for pemphigoid gestationis. It should be provided by an expert.
- Oral lesions are rare and usually follow skin eruptions.
- Oral lesions usually respond soon to the treatment.
- Corticosteroids are the mainstay of the treatment.
- Although most cases remit within 6 months of delivery, some are persistent.

Suggested Therapies

Systemic Treatment

Oral corticosteroids, prednisone or prednisolone, are the drugs of choice for pemphigoid gestationis. A dose of 20–60 mg/day, depending on the severity of the disease, usually achieves control of the disease and then the dose can be tapered to 10 mg/day or less, which can be slowly withdrawn. Systemic corticosteroids during the second and third trimester do not appear to place the fetus in danger.

Topical Treatment

Topical corticosteroids or antihistamines may be used for mild cases.

Alternative Therapies

Plasmapheresis should be used only in patients with severe disease and in whom systemic corticosteroids are contraindicated.

References

Chen SH, Chopra K, Evans TY, et al. Herpes gestationis in a mother and child. *J Am Acad Dermatol* 1999;40:847–849.

Jenkins R, Hern S, Black M. Clinical features and management of 87 patients with pemphigoid gestationis. *Clin Exp Dermatol* 1999;24:255–259.

Shimanovich I, Skrobek C, Rose C, et al. Pemphigoid gestationis with predominant involvement of oral mucous membranes and IgA autoantibodies targeting the C-terminus of BP180. *J Am Acad Dermatol* 2002;47:780–784.

Shornick JK, Bangert JL, Freeman RG, Gilliam JN. Herpes gestationis: Clinical and histologic features of twenty-eight cases. *J Am Acad Dermatol* 1983;8:214–224.

Triffet MK, Gibson LE, Leiferman KM. Severe subepidermal blistering disorder with features of bullous pemphigoid and herpes gestationis. *J Am Acad Dermatol* 1999;40:797–801.

Wojnarowska F, Kirtschig G, Khumalo N. Treatment of subepidermal immunobullous diseases. *Clin Dermatol* 2001;19:768–777.

Pemphigus

▨ Definition

Pemphigus is a group of chronic, bullous muco-cutaneous diseases that often primarily involve the oral mucosa.

▨ Etiology

Pemphigus is an autoimmune disorder. Desmosomal proteins desmoglein 3 (Dsg3) and desmoglein 1 (Dsg1) are the main targets of the immune response autoantigens. The clinical phenotype of pemphigus is determined by the underlying Dsg antibody profile and by the tissue distribution of Dsg1 and Dsg3. Mucosal pemphigus is usually seen in patients with Dsg3 antibodies.

▨ Classification

There are seven types of pemphigus based on clinical, histologic, and immunologic criteria:
- Pemphigus vulgaris (representing over 95% of all types)
- Pemphigus vegetans
- Pemphigus foliaceus
- Pemphigus erythematosus
- IgA pemphigus
- Drug-induced pemphigus
- Paraneoplastic pemphigus

▨ Main Clinical Features

The oral mucosa is mainly affected in pemphigus vulgaris. In 70–75% of cases, the primary manifestations of the disease occur in the oral mucosa. Almost all patients exhibit oral lesions at some stage of the disease.

Oral Mucosa

- Erythema, formation of bullae that rapidly rupture resulting in painful erosions. The lesions persist and progressively increase in number and size. The Nikolsky sign is positive. Soft palate, buccal mucosa, tongue, gingiva, and lips are the sites more frequently affected.

Other Mucosae

Conjunctiva, larynx, pharynx, esophagus, nose, genital, and rectal mucosa

Skin

Bullae that rupture easily leaving painful erosions that exhibit a tendency to increase in size. The trunk, scalp, umbilicus, and the intertriginous regions are more frequently affected.

▨ Diagnosis

The clinical diagnosis should be confirmed by histopathologic examination and direct and indirect immunofluorescent tests. The Tzanck smear test may also be helpful.

▨ Differential Diagnosis

- Cicatricial pemphigoid
- Bullous pemphigoid
- Linear IgA disease
- Pemphigoid gestationis
- Epidermolysis bullosa acquisita
- Dermatitis herpetiformis
- Erosive and bullous lichen planus
- Chronic ulcerative stomatitis
- Aphthous ulcers
- Behçet disease
- Herpes simplex
- Erythema multiforme
- Toxic epidermal necrolysis
- Drug-induced oral ulceration

▨ Treatment

Basic Guidelines

- The management of pemphigus is one of the most difficult problems in the field of dermatology and oral medicine and it should be undertaken only by specialists with extensive experience in managing the disease.
- Therapeutic regimens are dictated by the age of the patient, the degree of involvement, the

rate of disease progression, and the type of pemphigus.

- Pemphigus requires systemic therapy as early in the disease as possible.
- Systemic corticosteroids remain the therapeutic staple for pemphigus and have resulted in a dramatic drop in mortality.
- The high dosage and prolonged administration of corticosteroids often required to control the disease result in numerous side effects, many of which are serious or even life-threatening.
- Adjuvant therapies have been suggested to reduce the need for steroids.
- Topical treatment is only adjunctive in pemphigus treatment.
- Pemphigus vulgaris, pemphigus vegetans, and paraneoplastic pemphigus are more severe and resistant to treatment.
- Patients with severe cases of pemphigus must be hospitalized. Oral lesions are more resistant to treatment compared with skin lesions.

Suggested Therapies

Systemic Treatment

Corticosteroids

Systemic corticosteroids (prednisone or prednisolone) are the drugs of choice in patients with pemphigus. There are several strategies regarding the initial dose of treatment which may range between 0.5 mg/kg per day to 3 mg/kg per day. In our experience, the initial dose of prednisone or prednisolone should be flexible and should be customized to the individual needs of each patient depending on the severity of the disease. For example, patients with mild lesions may be treated initially with 50 mg/day for 2–3 weeks. Patients who do not respond to this treatment regimen or those who present initially with severe or rapidly progressive lesions should be treated with 80–120 mg/day or more until disease activity is controlled. The disease is thought to be clinically controlled when old lesions have healed and new lesions are absent. The dose that achieves clinical control of the disease is maintained for 2–3 weeks and then gradually tapered by 30% every 2 weeks until the dose of 20 mg/day is reached while maintaining clinical disease control. The dosage may subsequently be continued on alternate days and low-

ered by 5 mg every month until the dose of 5–10 mg every other day is achieved over a long period of time (1–3 years). Cessation of all treatment remains a judgment call for every physician.

Adjuvant Therapies

As a rule, adjuvant therapies should be used almost exclusively in combination with corticosteroids and rarely, if ever, as monotherapy for controlled cases of pemphigus. The reasons for using adjuvant therapies in pemphigus are: a) to reduce the need for corticosteroids, and hence their side effects, and b) to achieve better control of the disease. Depending on the mechanism of action, adjuvant therapies of pemphigus can be classified into three categories:

- immunosuppressive drugs (azathioprine, mycophenolate mofetil, cyclophosphamide, cyclosporine, and methotrexate)
- anti-inflammatory drugs (gold, dapsone, antimalarial drugs, tetracycline, nicotinamide)
- immunomodulatory procedures (plasmapheresis, extracorporeal photochemotherapy).

Azathioprine in a dose of 100 mg/day and mycophenolate mofetil in a dose of 2–3 g/day are the major immunosuppressive agents currently used more frequently. Plasmapheresis is indicated in very severe cases or cases resistant to corticosteroids.

Pulse Therapy

Pulse therapy refers to the discontinuous i.v. infusion of very high doses (megadoses) of corticosteroids (dexamethasone or methylprednisolone) and cyclophosphamide over a short period. This regimen must be used only in very severe cases and only in a hospital setting because it is associated with high morbidity and mortality.

Topical Treatment

Painful, resistant localized oral lesions may require the use of topical corticosteroids either in the form of a paste (0.1% triamcinolone acetonide in Orabase, or 0.05% clobetasol propionate gel) or in the form of intralesional injection every 2 weeks until the lesions heal. Topical corticosteroid therapy alone in insufficient for sustained control of the disease, as pemphigus is a systemic autoimmune disease and lesions will develop as long as there are adequate amounts of circulating pemphigus antibodies. Topical cyclosporine has also been used for oral lesions of pemphigus with partial success.

Future Therapies

Future therapies of pemphigus might be directed towards inducing compensating desmoglein isoforms.

References

Bystryn J-C, Steinman NM. The adjuvant therapy of pemphigus. *Arch Dermatol* 1996;132:203–212.

Enk AH, Knop J. Mycophenolate is effective in the treatment of pemphigus vulgaris. *Arch Dermatol* 1999;135:54–56.

Gooptu C, Staughton RCD. Use of topical cyclosporin in oral pemphigus. *J Am Acad Dermatol* 1998;38:860–861.

Grundmann-Kollmann M, Korting CH, Behrens S, et al. Mycophenolate mofetil: A new therapeutic option in the treatment of blistering autoimmune diseases. *J Am Acad Dermatol* 1999;40:957–960.

Harman KE, Seed PT, Bhogal BS, et al. The severity of cutaneous and oral pemphigus is related to desmoglein 1 and 3 antibody levels. *Br J Dermatol* 2001;144:775–780.

Korman NJ. New immunomodulating drugs in autoimmune blistering diseases. *Dermatol Clin* 2001;19:637–648.

Mignogna MD, Muzio LL, Mignogna RE, et al. Oral pemphigus: Long term behaviour and clinical response to treatment with deflazacort in sixteen cases. *J Oral Pathol Med* 2000;29:145–152.

Nousari HC, Anhalt GJ. The role of mycophenolate mofetil in the management of pemphigus. *Arch Dermatol* 1999;135:853–854.

Popovsky JL, Camisa C. New and emerging therapies for diseases of the oral cavity. *Dermatol Clin* 2000;18:113–125.

Stanley JR. Therapy of pemphigus vulgaris. *Arch Dermatol* 1999;135:76–78.

Stanley JR. Pathophysiology and therapy of pemphigus in the 21st century. *J Dermatol* 2001;28:645–646.

Veraldi S, Bocor M, Sarchi G, Caputo R. Treatment of pemphigus vulgaris with cyclosporine. *J Dermatol Treat* 1997;8:119–122.

Pericoronitis

Definition

Pericoronitis is an inflammatory reaction of the operculum covering an erupting or impacted tooth, usually the lower third molar.

Etiology

Trauma, accumulation of bacteria and debris beneath an operculum result in pericoronitis.

Main Clinical Features

- Redness and swelling of the operculum and gingiva
- Ulcerated operculum and abscess formation
- Pain, trismus, halitosis
- Occasionally low-grade fever
- Regional lymphadenopathy
- Malaise

Diagnosis

The diagnosis is exclusively based on the symptoms and clinical presentation. Radiographs may be useful.

Differential Diagnosis

- Necrotizing ulcerative gingivitis
- Herpetic gingivitis
- Leukemia
- Infectious mononucleosis
- Pemphigus
- Cicatricial pemphigoid
- Non-Hodgkin lymphoma

Treatment

Basic Guidelines

- A high level of oral hygiene is always recommended to avoid recurrences.

- When the acute phase has subsided the operculum or the impacted tooth should be removed.

Suggested Therapies

Topical Treatment

Acute pericoronitis is treated with gentle topical use of antiseptics (chlorhexidine or oxygenating agents). Remove the food debris, bacteria, or any other irritation underneath the gingival flap (operculum) and irrigate with saline. Gentle application of 50% trichloracetic acid to the undersurface of the operculum results in immediate cessation of pain.

Systemic Treatment

Systemic use of antibiotics such as metronidazole 250–500 mg three times daily for 4–6 days or erythromycin 500 mg/day for 4–6 days or penicillin 1–2 MIU/day for 4–5 days is indicated if there are systemic signs and symptoms.

Surgical removal of the operculum or/and extraction of the offending tooth after the acute phase has subsided is recommended to avoid recurrences.

References

Bataineh AB, Ai QM. The predisposing factors of pericoronitis of mandibular third molars in a Jordanian population. *Quintessence Int* 2003;34:227–231.

Laine M, Venta I, Hyrkas T, et al. Chronic inflammatory around painless partially erupted third molars. *Oral Surg Oral Med Oral Pathol Oral Radiol Endod* 2003;95: 277–282.

Orbak R, Dayi E. Flow-cytometric analysis of T-lymphocyte subset after different treatment methods in patients with pericoronitis. *J Oral Maxillofac Surg* 2003;61:201–205.

Sixou JL, Magaud C, Jolivet-Gougeon A, et al. Microbiology of mandibular third molar pericoronitis: Incidence of betalactamase-producing bacteria. *Oral Surg Oral Med Oral Pathol Oral Radiol Endod* 2003;95:655–659.

Peripheral Facial Nerve Paralysis

▧ Definition

Peripheral facial nerve paralysis or Bell palsy is an acute idiopathic unilateral facial paresis of the lower motor neuron type.

▧ Etiology

The etiology is unknown. However, a viral etiology (herpes simplex virus, varicella-zoster virus) is possible.

▧ Main Clinical Features

- Acute, unilateral abrupt-onset facial paresis
- Dropping of the angle of the mouth of the involved side and inability to close the eyelid, or to grin, or to whistle are characteristic features
- Additional common symptoms are disturbances in taste and mastication, pain around the angle of the jaw on the affected side, pain and numbness of the ear, reduced lacrimation
- More common in young and middle-aged individuals

▧ Diagnosis

The diagnosis is based on the clinical features. However, electrodiagnostic tests may be helpful.

▧ Differential Diagnosis

- Lyme disease
- Melkersson–Rosenthal syndrome
- Heerfordt syndrome
- Angioedema
- Peripheral facial paresis due to parotid tumors
- Peripheral facial paresis due to systemic diseases

▧ Treatment

Basic Guidelines

- All patients with acute facial palsy require a full neurologic evaluation before the diagnosis of Bell palsy is made.
- Most patients (50–60%) with peripheral facial nerve paralysis recover completely without treatment, particularly those with mild disease.
- All patients should be provided protection for the eyes by an ophthalmologist for the duration of the disease.
- The management of Bell palsy should be undertaken by a neurologist.

Suggested Therapies

- Oral prednisone 50–80 mg/day is the drug of choice in two divided doses for 5–10 days, followed by tapering the dose and stopping it in the next 8–12 days. The efficacy of corticosteroids is related to early treatment, and the dose. However, the efficacy of corticosteroids treatment has been questioned by some physicians.
- Oral acyclovir or valacyclovir in combination with prednisone have been used with success.

References

Eidlitz-Markus T, Gilai A, Mimuni M, Shuper A. Recurrent facial nerve palsy in paediatric patients. *Eur J Pediatr* 2001;160:659–663.

Peitersen E. Natural history of Bell's palsy. *Acta Otolaryngol Suppl* 1992;492:122.

Peitersen E. Bell's palsy: The spontaneous course of 2500 peripheral facial nerve palsies of different etiologies. *Acta Otolaryngol Suppl* 2002;549:4–30.

Plasma Cell Cheilitis

Definition

Plasma cell cheilitis is an uncommon inflammatory disorder of the lips characterized by dense infiltration of mature plasma cells.

Etiology

The etiology is unknown, although an allergic reaction to gum chewing and dentifrice products have been thought to be responsible.

Main Clinical Features

- Diffuse erythema and mild swelling of the vermilion border of the lips, usually the lower lip
- A mild burning sensation may be present
- Similar lesions may occur on the gingiva and the tongue
- The lesions are identical to plasma cell balanitis/Zoon balanitis

Diagnosis

The clinical diagnosis should be confirmed by a biopsy and histopathologic examination.

Differential Diagnosis

- Contact cheilitis
- Cheilitis glandularis
- Actinic cheilitis
- Erythematous candidiasis
- Lichen planus
- Lupus erythematosus
- Erythroplakia

Treatment

Basic Guidelines

- Exclude any other causes of inflammation.
- The treatment is symptomatic as the exact cause is unclear.
- Discontinuation of gum chewing, dentifrices, and mouthwashes.

Suggested Therapies

- Low- or medium-potency topical corticosteroids twice daily for about 2–4 weeks may provide relief of erythema. However, recurrences are not unusual.
- Systemic oral corticosteroids, e.g., prednisone 10–20 mg/day for 2–3 weeks and then tapering the dose and discontinuation after about 2 weeks, may be used in persistent cases.

References

Baughman RD, Berger P, Pringle WM. Plasma cell cheilitis. *Arch Dermatol* 1974;110:725–726.

Silverman S Jr, Lozada F. An epilogue to plasma-cell gingivostomatitis (allergic gingivostomatitis). *Oral Surg Oral Med Oral Pathol* 1977;43:211–217.

Tamaki K, Osada A, Tsukamoto K, et al. Treatment of plasma cell cheilitis with griseofulvin. *J Am Acad Dermatol* 1995;33:319.

Yoganathan S, Bohn TG, Mason G. Plasma cell balanitis and vulvitis (of Zoon). A study of 10 cases. *J Reprod Med* 1994;39:939–944.

Plasminogen Deficiency: Gingival Lesions

▓ Definition

Gingival lesions due to plasminogen deficiency is a rare disorder due to fibrin deposition in the connective tissues.

▓ Etiology

It is an autosomal recessive disorder resulting in a defect in plasminogen function.

▓ Main Clinical Features

- Gingival overgrowth that is more severe in the interdental papillae
- Multiple superficial, painful gingival ulcerations covered by whitish-yellow pseudomembranes
- Ligneous conjunctivitis
- Rarely, lesions may develop in the larynx, nose, and cervix
- No tendency toward thrombosis

▓ Diagnosis

The clinical diagnosis should be confirmed by a biopsy and histopathologic examination and assay of plasma functional plasminogen activity.

▓ Differential Diagnosis

- Hereditary gingival fibromatosis
- Amyloidosis
- Lipoid proteinosis
- Hurler syndrome
- Other forms of mucopolysaccharidoses
- Crohn disease

▓ Treatment

Basic Guidelines

- A high level of oral hygiene should be maintained.

- Avoid toothbrushing with a hard toothbrush during the acute phase of the gingival lesions
- The treatment of ligneous conjunctivitis must be provided by an ophthalmologist.

Suggested Therapies

Topical Treatment

- Topical application of heparin two to three times daily for about 1 week.
- Topical application of corticosteroids in the form of 0.1 % triamcinolone acetonide in Orabase twice daily may prove useful for the gingival lesions by reducing inflammation and promoting healing.

Systemic Treatment

- Oral pentoxifylline 400 mg twice daily for 6–10 days is very effective and helped the gingival ulceration to heal in my experience with two patients.
- Intravenous purified plasminogen concentrate may be used in severe plasminogen deficiency, but only by a specialist.

References

Gokbuget AY, Mutlu S, Scully C, et al. Amyloidaceous ulcerated gingival hyperplasia: A newly described entity related to ligneous conjunctivitis. *J Oral Pathol Med* 1997;26:100–104.

Laskaris G, Scully C. *Periodontal Manifestations of Local and Systemic Diseases.* Springer Verlag: Berlin, 2003.

Scully C, Gokbuget AY, Allen C, et al. Oral lesions indicative of plasminogen deficiency (hypoplasminogenemia). *Oral Surg Oral Med Oral Pathol Oral Radiol Endod* 2001;91:334–337.

Suresh L, Aguirre A, Kumar V, et al. Recurrent recalcitrant gingival hyperplasia and plasminogen deficiency: A case report. *J Periodontol* 2003;74:1508–1513.

Pyostomatitis Vegetans

Definition

Pyostomatitis vegetans is a rare pustular disorder of the oral mucosa associated with inflammatory bowel diseases, particularly ulcerative colitis and Crohn disease.

Etiology

The etiology is unknown.

Main Clinical Features

Pyostomatitis vegetans is believed to be the oral equivalent of pyodermatitis vegetans of the skin.

- Multiple, usually painless, yellow-white, soft vegetative mucosal folds that contain pustular microabscesses
- Microabscesses progressively result in erosions or ulcerations
- Red oral mucosa
- Buccal and labial mucosa, gingiva, soft palate, and tongue are more frequently affected

Diagnosis

The clinical diagnosis should be confirmed by a biopsy and histopathologic examination.

Differential Diagnosis

- Pemphigus vegetans
- Dermatitis herpetiformis
- Herpetic gingivostomatitis
- Herpangina
- Crohn disease
- Herpetiform ulcers

Treatment

Basic Guidelines

- Before treatment medical evaluation by a specialist for the possibility of bowel disease is necessary.
- Appropriate management of the bowel disease usually results in regression of the concomitant oral lesions.
- A combination of systemic and local treatment is necessary for a permanent cure.

Suggested Therapies

- Systemic corticosteroids, e.g., prednisone 30–60 mg/day for about 1–2 weeks and then tapering the dose to a maintenance dose of 5–10 mg/day for 1–2 months, control the disease.
- Sulfasalazine 1–1.5 g twice daily is an alternative second-line regimen, particularly in patients who have associated ulcerative colitis and Crohn disease.
- Topical corticosteroids such as clobetasol, triamcinolone, or fluocinonide may be helpful.

References

Chan SWY, Scully C, Prime SS, Eveson J. Pyostomatitis vegetans: Oral manifestations of ulcerative colitis. *Oral Surg Oral Med Oral Pathol* 1991;72:689–692.

Ficarra G, Amorosi A, Piluso SP. Oral Crohn's disease and pyostomatitis vegetans: An unusual presentation. *Oral Surg Oral Med Oral Pathol Oral Radiol Endod* 1993;75: 220–224.

Gionchetti P, Rizello F, Habal F, et al. Standard treatment of ulcerative colitis. *Dig Dis* 2003;21:157–167.

Neville BW, Laden SA, Smith SE, et al. Pyostomatitis vegetans. *Am J Dermatopathol* 1985;7:69–77.

Thornbill MH, Zakrzewska JM, Gilkes JJH. Pyostomatitis vegetans: Report of three cases and review of the literature. *J Oral Pathol Med* 1992;21:128–133.

Radiation-Induced Oral Mucositis

▓ Definition

Radiation-induced oral mucositis is one of the most common toxicities related to head and neck cancer radiotherapy.

▓ Etiology

The mucositis occurs as a side effect of radiation.

▓ Main Clinical Features

Radiation oral mucositis usually appears during the second week of radiotherapy.

- Erythema and edema of the oral mucosa are early signs that appear at the end of the first week of the radiotherapy
- Erosions and ulcerations covered by a whitish pseudomembranous exudate develop during the second week
- Burning sensation, pain, loss of taste, and xerostomia are common
- Lesions persist during the period of treatment and for some weeks thereafter

▓ Diagnosis

The diagnosis is based on the medical history and the clinical features.

▓ Differential Diagnosis

- Mucositis due to chemotherapy
- Graft-versus-host disease
- Erythema multiforme
- Erosive lichen planus
- Cicatricial pemphigoid
- Bullous pemphigoid
- Pemphigus
- Herpetic stomatitis
- Leukemia
- Allergic contact stomatitis

▓ Treatment

Basic Guidelines

- Pretreatment eradication of infection and maintenance of high level of oral hygiene is important before radiotherapy. Periodontal and dental treatment must be done before cancer therapy.
- Patients should be advised to avoid the use of tobacco and alcohol.
- Radiation therapy breaks are necessary if the oral mucositis is severe.
- The severity of oral mucositis is related to the field and the dose of radiation.
- Mild mucositis may resolve 2–4 weeks after cessation of radiotherapy

Suggested Therapies

Topical Treatment

- Topical anesthetics (e.g., viscous lidocaine), topical corticosteroid ointment in Orabase, or tacrolimus ointment and antimicrobial lozenges have been used with limited success.
- 0.15 % benzydamine oral rinse has also been used for prophylactic treatment of radiation-induced mucositis.
- Topical mouthwashes with GM-CSF and sucralfate have also been used unsuccessfully.

Systemic Treatment

- Systemic corticosteroids in low doses, e.g., prednisone 15–20 mg/day for 2–3 weeks are very effective and relief the symptoms and signs of severe oral mucositis dramatically. High doses of B-complex vitamins in combination with corticosteroids are also helpful.
- Oral zinc sulfate supplementation is beneficial in decreasing the severity of radiation-induced oral mucositis.
- Chemical radioprotection using amifostine has recently been approved for use in head and neck cancer to protect against radiation-induced mucositis and salivary gland dysfunction.

References

Andreassen CN, Grau C, Lindegaard JC. Chemical radioprotection: A critical review of amifostine as a cytoprotector in radiotherapy. *Semin Radiat Oncol* 2003;13:62–72.

Dodd MJ, Miaskowski C, Greenspan D, et al. Radiation-induced mucositis: A randomized clinical trial of micronized sucralfate versus salt and soda mouthwashes. *Cancer Invest* 2003;21:21–33.

Epstein JB, Silverman S Jr, Paggiarino DA, et al. Benzydamine HCL for prophylaxis of radiation-induced oral mucositis: Results from a multicenter, randomized, double-blind, placebo-controlled clinical trial. *Curr Oncol Rep* 2002;4:65–66.

Ertekin MV, Koc M, Karslioglu I, Sezen O. Zinc sulfate in the prevention of radiation-induced oropharyngeal mucositis: a prospective, placebo-controlled randomized study. *Int J Radiat Oncol Biol Phys* 2004;58:167–174.

Johnson JT. Prevention of radiation-induced mucositis. *Curr Oncol Rep* 2001;3:56–58.

Lapeyere M, Charra-Brunaud C, Kaminsky MC, et al. Management of mucositis following radiotherapy for head and neck cancers. *Cancer Radiother* 2001;1(suppl 1):121S–130S.

Plevova P. Preventing and treatment of chemotherapy and radiotherapy-induced oral mycositis: A review. *Oral Oncol* 1999;35:453–470.

Saarilahti K, Jakanti M, Joensuu T, et al. Comparison of granulocyte-macrophage colony-stimulating factor and sucralfate mouthwashes in the protection of radiation-induced mycositis: A double-blind prospective randomized phase III study. *Int J Radiat Oncol Biol Phys* 2002;54:479–485.

Sarcoidosis

■ Definition

Sarcoidosis is a multisystemic granulomatous disease with a broad spectrum of clinical expression.

■ Etiology

The etiology is unknown. One hypothesis is that *Mycobacterium tuberculosis* and other Mycobacteria species may play a role in the pathogenesis. An immune response may lead to granuloma formation.

■ Main Clinical Features

The disease affects the lungs, lymph nodes, liver, spleen, bones, eyes, nervous system, skin, salivary glands, and rarely the oral mucosa. Some patients are asymptomatic.

Oral Lesions

- Small or large red nodules or plaques, which rarely ulcerate
- Loosening of teeth
- Temporomandibular joint disfunction
- Bilateral major salivary gland and regional lymph node enlargement and eye involvement (Heerfordt syndrome)
- The lips, tongue, and gingiva are most frequently affected

Skin Lesions

- Multiple purple-brown macules, papules, or nodules
- Lupus pernio, erythema nodosum, scars
- Symmetrical purple plaques with telangiectasia
- Skin lesions occur in 25–30% of patients and may be the only manifestations

Other Organ Involvement

- Eyes (uveitis, iridocyclitis)
- Lungs
- Bones (arthralgia, multiple cysts in distal phalanges)

- Hepatosplenomegaly
- Lymphadenopathy
- Central nervous system involvement, diabetes insipidus
- Heart and larynx

Constitutional Symptoms

- Fever
- Malaise
- Dyspnea

■ Diagnosis

The clinical diagnosis should be confirmed by a biopsy and histopathologic examination, chest radiography, elevated serum angiotensin-converting enzyme (ACE) levels, bone radiographs, and serum calcium levels.

■ Differential Diagnosis

- Tuberculosis
- Crohn disease
- Amyloidosis
- Erythematous candidiasis
- Non-Hodgkin lymphoma
- Leishmaniasis
- Syphilis
- Erythroplakia

■ Treatment

Basic Guidelines

- Systemic treatment of sarcoidosis is reserved for patients with systemic signs and symptoms.
- The treatment of oral lesions is part of the therapy for the systemic disease.
- The choice of drugs, the dose and duration of therapy are dependent on the organs involved and the severity of the disease.
- The treatment of sarcoidosis must be provided by a specialist.

Suggested Therapies

- Systemic corticosteroids are the cornerstone of therapy for sarcoidosis. Prednisone 40–60 mg/day for 4–6 weeks then tapered for a total course of 12–24 months.
- Immunosuppressive drugs such as azathioprine, cyclosporine, methotrexate, and cyclophosphamide are alternative therapeutic agents.
- Antimalarials, thalidomide, pentoxifylline, and allopurinol have also been used as second-line agents with partial success.
- Infliximab and etanercept are tumor necrosis factor alpha blockers and have recently been used with success in the therapy of resistant sarcoidosis.
- Topical or intralesional corticosteroids are the treatment of choice for cutaneous and oral lesions.

References

Batal H, Chou LL, Cottrell DA. Sarcoidosis. Medical and dental implications. *Oral Surg Oral Med Oral Pathol Oral Radiol Endod* 1999;88:386.

James DG, Sharma OP. Parotid gland sarcoidosis. *Sarcoidosis Vasc Diffuse Lung Dis* 2000;17:27–32.

Newman L, Rose C, Maier L. Sarcoidosis. *N Engl J Med* 1997; 336:1224–1234.

Reich JM. Adverse long-term effect of corticosteroid therapy in recent onset sarcoidosis. *Sarcoidosis Vasc Diffuse Lung Dis* 2003;20:227–234.

Reimold AM. TNF alpha as therapeutic target: new drugs, more applications. *Curr Drug Targets Inflamm Allergy* 2002;1:377–392.

Tong Z, Dai H, Chen B, et al. Inhibition of cytokine release from alveolar macrophages in pulmonary sarcoidosis by pentoxifylline: Comparison with dexamethasone. *Chest* 2003;124:1526–1532.

Ulbricht KU, Stoll M, Bierwirth J, et al. Successful tumor necrosis factor alpha blockade treatment in therapy-resistant sarcoidosis. *Arthritis Rheum* 2003;48:3542–3543.

Walter MC, Lochmuller H, Schloffer-Weigel B, et al. Successful treatment of muscle sarcoidosis with thalidomide. *Acta Myol* 2003;22:22–25.

Sarcomas

■ Definition

Oral sarcomas are a rare group of malignant neoplasms originating from the oral mesenchymal cells.

■ Etiology

The etiology is unknown.

■ Classification

- Fibrosarcoma
- Malignant fibrous histiocytoma
- Neurofibrosarcoma
- Liposarcoma
- Malignant hemangioendothelioma
- Malignant hemangiopericytoma
- Angiosarcoma
- Kaposi sarcoma
- Leiomyosarcoma
- Rhabdomyosarcoma
- Alveolar soft part sarcoma
- Osteosarcoma
- Chondrosarcoma
- Ewing sarcoma

■ Main Clinical Features

Almost all oral sarcomas presents with similar clinical signs and symptoms.

- Painless or painful, rapidly or slowly growing swelling or mass
- The mass may be soft or semi-hard or hard on palpation with or without ulceration
- The color may be red, blue red, or normal
- The tongue, palate, buccal mucosa, gingiva, and the jaws are more frequently affected
- Bony swelling, loosening of teeth, and paresthesia are common in jaws sarcomas

■ Diagnosis

The clinical diagnosis should be confirmed by biopsy and histopathologic examination.

■ Differential Diagnosis

- Soft tissue sarcomas
- Soft tissue abscess
- Pyogenic granuloma
- Hemangioma
- Peripheral giant cell granuloma
- Non-Hodgkin lymphoma
- Salivary gland tumors
- Squamous cell carcinoma

■ Treatment

Basic Guidelines

- Before treatment an accurate diagnosis should be made.
- A follow-up program should be suggested to the patients because the rate of recurrence chances of metastasis are high.
- Details of the treatment modalities are beyond the scope of this book.

Suggested Therapies

- Radical surgical excision is the treatment of choice for the great majority of oral sarcomas.
- Radiotherapy is the second line of treatment, usually in conjunction with surgery and chemotherapy.
- Systemic chemotherapy may be helpful, usually in conjunction with surgery and radiotherapy.
- Intralesional injection of vinblastine may be used with success for the treatment of individual oral lesions of Kaposi sarcoma.
- Because of multifocality of Kaposi sarcoma, treatment with chemotherapy and/or radiotherapy is favored over surgery.

References

Antman K, Chang Y. Kaposi's sarcoma. *N Engl J Med* 2000; 342:1027–1038.

Dezube BJ. AIDS-related Kaposi's sarcoma: The role of local therapy for a systemic disease. *Arch Dermatol* 2000;136: 1554–1556.

Fielding AF, Lindemeyer R, Wood-Harris J, Hartman MJ. Ewing sarcoma of the mandible: A combined approach to treatment. *J Clin Pediatr Dent* 2002;26:409–412.

Fonseca RJ. *Oral and Maxillofacial Surgery. Surgical Pathology*, Vol. 5. WB Saunders Co: Philadelphia, 2000.

Gascon P, Schwartz RA. Kaposi's sarcoma. New treatment modalities. *Dermatol Clin* 2000;18:169–175.

Jordan RC, Regezi JA. Oral spindle cell neoplams: A review of 307 cases. *Oral Surg Oral Med Oral Pathol Oral Radiol Endod* 2003;95:717–724.

Laskaris G. *Color Atlas of Oral Diseases*, 3rd edition. Thieme Verlag: Stuttgart, 2003.

Nikitakis NG, Lopes MA, Razoki AE, et al. Oral liposarcoma: Case report and review of the literature. *Oral Surg Oral Med Oral Pathol Oral Radiol Endod* 2001;92:194–201.

Nikitakis NG, Lopes MA, Bailey JS, et al. Oral leiomyosarcoma: Review of the literature and report of two cases with assessment of the prognostic and diagnostic significance of immunohistochemical and molecular markers. *Oral Oncol* 2002;38:201–208.

Ramirez-Amador V, Esquivel-Pedraza L, Lozada-Nur F, et al. Intralesional vinblastine vs 3 % sodium tetradecyl sulfate for the treatment of oral Kaposi's sarcoma: A double blind, randomized clinical trial. *Oral Oncol* 2002;38: 460–467.

Randey M, Thomas G, Mathew A, et al. Sarcoma of the oral and maxillofacial soft tissue in adults. *Eur J Surg Oncol* 2000;26:145–148.

Scleroderma

▪ Definition

Scleroderma is a multisystemic, chronic disorder characterized by immune activation and diffuse fibrosis of the skin and internal organs.

▪ Etiology

The etiology is unknown. However, autoimmunity and fibroblast dysregulation play an important role in the pathogenesis of the disease.

▪ Classification

There are two main types of scleroderma: localized (morphea) and systemic.

▪ Main Clinical Features

The oral mucosa is only involved in systemic scleroderma and the lesions usually follow the other systemic manifestations.

Oral Manifestations

Pale and thin oral mucosa, atrophy and smooth dorsal surface of the tongue, disappearance of the palatal folds, and a short and inelastic lingual frenum, which may result in dysarthria. Tongue induration, ulcers on the oral mucosa, and microstomia may occur. In 20% of cases widening of the periodontal space is seen on radiographs

Skin Manifestations

Subcutaneous edema, telangiectasia, pigmentation, depigmentation, and subcutaneous calcification are common. The skin progressively becomes thickened and inelastic with loss of normal folds. Raynaud's phenomenon is common and an early manifestation. Ulcers, usually on the finger tips, may be seen

Gastrointestinal Manifestations

Dysphagia due to esophageal dysfunction, and fibrosis and atrophy of the gastrointestinal tract leading to hypomotility and malabsorption

Pulmonary Manifestations

Pulmonary fibrosis and vascular disease are common

Cardiac Manifestations

Pericarditis, cardiomyopathy, arrhythmia, and heart block may occur

Renal Manifestations

Renal failure leading to a rapidly progressive syndrome of hypertension

▪ Diagnosis

The clinical diagnosis should be confirmed by histopathologic examination and positive tests to antinuclear (ANA) and SCL-70 antibodies.

▪ Differential Diagnosis

- Oral submucous fibrosis
- Cicatricial pemphigoid
- Lipoid proteinosis
- Epidermolysis bullosa
- Porphyria cutanea tarda
- Systemic lupus erythematosus
- Dermatomyositis
- Eosinophilic fasciitis

▪ Treatment

Basic Guidelines

- The treatment of scleroderma is difficult and remains a great challenge for the clinician. It should be provided by specialists (rheumatologist, dermatologist, and internist). The role of the stomatologist is mainly geared to the prevention and treatment of the oral complications.
- Maintenance of excellent oral hygiene is recommended to prevent tooth loss and periodontal disease.
- Efforts should be made to determine the activity of the disease process and the degree of

specific organ involvement before specific treatment decisions are made.

- Therapies are directed to:
  — improve peripheral blood circulation with vasodilators and antiplatelet aggregation drugs
  — prevent the synthesis and release of harmful cytokines with immunosuppressant drugs, and
  — reduce or inhibit fibrosis with agents that reduce collagen synthesis or enhance collagenase production.

Suggested Therapies

- Vasodilators (calcium channel blockers), pentoxifylline, angiotensin-converting enzyme inhibitors, and prostaglandins.
- Immunosuppressant drugs such as cyclophosphamide, cyclosporine, methotrexate, and extracorporeal photopheresis.
- Antifibrinolytic agents such as D-penicillamine, colchicine, interferon gamma, and relaxin.
- Corticosteroids (prednisolone) are the most effective drugs in the early inflammatory stage and can be used in association with other immunosuppressants.

- PUVA (psoralen and ultraviolet radiation) bath photochemotherapy.
- Surgical correction of oral complications such as the short and inelastic lingual frenum and microstomia.

Alternative and Future Therapies

Thalidomide, minocycline, statins, anti-integrins, anti-transforming growth factor-beta, autologous stem cell transplantation, and transplantation have been suggested.

References

Bridges MJ, Kelly CA. Raynaud's phenomenon affecting the tongue of a patient with scleroderma. *Ann Rheum Dis* 2002;61:472.

Sapadin AN, Fleischmajer R. Treatment of scleroderma. *Arch Dermatol* 2002;138:99–105.

Steen VD. Treatment of systemic sclerosis. *Am J Clin Dermatol* 2001;2:315–325.

Sule SD, Wigley FM. Treatment of scleroderma: an update. *Expert Opin Invest Drugs* 2003;12:471–482.

Terzoglu A, Cigsar B, Aslan G. Surgical correction of microstomia in a patient with scleroderma. *Ann Plast Surg* 2002;49:222–223.

Scurvy

■ Definition

Scurvy is a rare disease due to vitamin C deficiency leading to reduction of collagen synthesis and capillary fragility with hemorrhages and poor wound healing due to the vessel weakness.

■ Etiology

The cause is vitamin C (ascorbic acid) deficiency. In present times the deficiency is limited to individuals whose diets are poor in fresh fruits and vegetables.

■ Main Clinical Features

The gingiva and the oral mucosa are frequently affected.

Oral Manifestations

- Generalized gingival swelling and redness
- Spontaneous gingival hemorrhage and ulcerations, tooth mobility, and periodontal bone loss are common
- Oral mucosal petechiae, hemorrhages, ecchymoses, and delayed wound healing are also common
- Enamel hypoplasia of the developing teeth may occur

Other Manifestations

- Follicular hyperkeratosis, skin hemorrhages, and ecchymoses
- Conjunctival hemorrhages, melena, hematuria, and subperiosteal hemorrhages are common
- There may be tenderness of the lower limbs and inability to walk
- Moderate to severe anemia
- Subarachnoid and intracerebral hemorrhages may occur in untreated cases
- Weakness, fatigue, weight loss, lassitude

■ Diagnosis

The clinical diagnosis may be confirmed by decreased serum ascorbic acid levels (usually below 0.1 mg/dL).

■ Differential Diagnosis

- Necrotizing ulcerative gingivitis
- Primary herpetic gingivostomatitis
- Thrombocytopenic purpura
- Agranulocytosis
- Aplastic anemia
- Leukemia
- Protein deficiency

■ Treatment

Basic Guidelines

- A diet rich in fresh fruits and vegetables should be ensured.
- Improve oral hygiene.

Suggested Therapies

- Oral administration of ascorbic acid 1–2 g/day improves the patient's condition dramatically and all signs and symptoms soon disappear.
- Topical mouthwashes with oxygen-releasing agents, e.g., carbamide peroxide, several times daily is helpful for the oral lesions.
- A plaque control program should be followed.

References

Christopher K, Tammaro D, Wing EJ. Early scurvy complication anorexia nerosa. *South Med J* 2002;95:1065–1066.

Oeffinger KC. Scurvy: More than historical relevance. *Am Fam Phys* 1993;48:609–613.

Ratanachu-Ek S, Sukswai P, Jeerathanyasakun Y, Wongtapradit L. Scurvy in pediatric patients: A review of 28 cases. *J Med Assoc Thai* 2003;86(suppl 3):S734–S740.

Sjögren Syndrome

Definition

Sjögren syndrome or autoimmune epitheliitis is a chronic autoimmune exocrinopathy that predominantly involves salivary, lacrimal, and other exocrine glands, resulting in decreased secretions.

Etiology

Sjögren syndrome is an autoimmune disorder.

Classification

- Primary: when the disease occurs alone
- Secondary: when the disease coexists with collagen diseases such as rheumatoid arthritis, systemic lupus erythematosus, scleroderma, polymyositis, Hashimoto thyroiditis, primary biliary cirrhosis, vasculitides, or cryoglobulinemia.

Main Clinical Features

The disease commonly effects women (ratio 9 : 1) mainly during the fourth and fifth decades of life and is usually benign. However, the quality of life is influenced by the nature of the associated disease. Approximately 5% of patients develop a non-Hodgkin B-cell lymphoma.

Oral Lesions

Recurrent enlargement of the parotids or other major and minor salivary glands, xerostomia and severe dental caries. Oral candidiasis, gingivitis, and cheilitis are common

Ocular Lesions

Keratoconjunctivitis sicca: in severe cases may lead to blindness
Desiccation may involve the nose, throat, larynx, bronchi, and vagina

Skin Lesions

Dry skin, purpura, annular erythema, Raynaud phenomenon, and pernio-like lesions may occur.

Extraglandular Lesions

Occur in about 30% of patients with primary disease and include fatigue, low-grade fever, myalgias, arthralgias, pancreatitis, pulmonary and renal involvement, chronic liver disease, vasculitis, and neurological dysfunction

Diagnosis

The clinical diagnosis should be confirmed by histopathologic examination of the labial minor salivary glands and positive serologic tests (ANA, anti-DNA antibodies, anti SS-A [Ro], SS-B [La], and rheumatoid factor).

Differential Diagnosis

- HIV infection
- Sarcoidosis
- Heerfordt syndrome
- Chronic graft-versus-host-disease
- Primary amyloidosis
- Systemic sclerosis
- Mikulicz syndrome
- Sialosis
- Xerostomia due to drugs and neurologic disorders
- Iron deficiency anemia

Treatment

Basic Guidelines

- The treatment of Sjögren syndrome is symptomatic and supportive as no therapeutic measures can significantly alter the course of the disease.
- Close collaboration between the rheumatologist, ophthalmologist, stomatologist, and dentist is necessary for the treatment of the patients.
- In secondary disease, the treatment of the associated disease should be carried out independently of the presence of Sjögren syndrome.

- A regimen of oral hygiene is important in order to preserve the dentition and to prevent periodontal disease.
- Patients should avoid drugs which cause xerostomia (anticholinergic, sympathomimetics, antidepressants etc) and smoking.

Suggested Therapies

Systemic Treatment

Oral Corticosteroids

Prednisolone 20–40 mg/day and immunosuppressive drugs (cyclophosphamide or azathioprine) have been used to control severe disease particularly with extraglandular involvement.

Hydroxychloroquine

Plaquenil 100–300 mg/day may be helpful in patients with extraglandular disease. However, it is usually not effective for oral and ocular dryness.

Stimulation of the residual exocrine glands can be achieved with systemic cholinergic parasympathomimetics such as pilocarpine hydrochloride (Salagen 5 mg tablet, three times daily). Recently, cevimeline hydrochloride (Evoxac 30 mg capsule three times daily), a muscarinic receptor agonist has been shown to increase salivary secretion and improved subjective and objective symptoms of patients with xerostomia in Sjögren syndrome. Neither of these drugs should be used in patients with narrow-angle glaucoma or iritis, uncontrolled asthma, heart failure, renal disease, chronic obstructive pulmonary disease, and pregnancy.

Topical Treatment

For symptomatic relief of xerostomia topical use of saliva substitutes (Salivart, Xero-Lube, Saliva Orthana, Oralbalance, Saliveze, Salivix) several times daily is recommended. Artificial tears, ophthalmic lubricants, and local stimulators of tear secretions are used for dryness of the eyes and must be given by the ophthalmologist.

Alternative Therapy

Sjögren syndrome is a new indication for TNF-alpha inhibitors use.

References

Ferguson MM. Pilocarpine and other cholinergic drugs in the management of salivary gland dysfunction. *Oral Surg Oral Med Oral Pathol* 1993;75:186–191.

Fife RS, Chase WF, Dore RK, et al. Cevimeline for the treatment of xerostomia in patients with Sjögren's syndrome: a randomized trial. *Arch Intern Med* 2002;162:1293–1300.

Mariette X. Current and potential treatments for primary Sjögren's syndrome. *Joint Bone Spine* 2002;69:363–366.

Moutsopoulos HM. Sjögren's syndrome-autoimmune epitheliitis. *Clin Immunol Immunopathol* 1994;72:162–165.

Rostron J, Rogers S, Longman L, et al. Health-related quality of life in patients with primary Sjögren's syndrome and xerostomia: A comparative study. *Gerodontology* 2002;19:53–59.

Shiozawa A. Cevimeline hydrochloride hydrate: A review of its pharmacological profiles and clinical potential in xerostomia [in Japanese]. *Nippon Yakurigaku Zasshi* 2002;120:253–258.

Talal N, Moutsopoulos HM, Kassan SS. *Sjögren's syndrome: Clinical and immunological aspects.* Springer Verlag: Berlin, 1987.

Smokeless Tobacco Keratosis

Definition

Smokeless tobacco keratosis is a white keratotic lesion of the mandibular vestibule encountered in users of smokeless tobacco or snuff.

Etiology

Mucosal contact with smokeless tobacco stored in the vestibular area.

Main Clinical Features

- Thin, gray-white translucent plaque that appears fissured or rippled
- It usually takes 1–5 years for the lesion to develop
- The white plaque may thicken gradually to the point of appearing nodular
- The lesion is usually confined to the area of placement of the smokeless tobacco, is painless, and does not detach
- Gingival recession and staining of the roots of the teeth in the area may be present as well

Diagnosis

The diagnosis is based on the history and the clinical features. Biopsy is occasionally necessary to rule out premalignant and malignant changes.

Differential Diagnosis

- Leukoplakia
- Squamous cell carcinoma
- Candidiasis
- Lichen planus
- White sponge nevus
- Cinnamon contact stomatitis

Treatment

Basic Guidelines

- If the lesion is not extensively thick and is histologically benign, habit cessation leads to reversal of the lesion within 2–6 weeks in the majority of smokeless tobacco users.
- After discontinuation of the smokeless tobacco habit, the lesion will diminish in size but will not disappear completely. Any lesion remaining after 6 weeks should be biopsied.

Suggested Therapies

- Smoking cessation.
- Surgical excision if the lesions persist.

References

Hirsch JM, Johansson SL. Effect of long-term application of snuff on the oral mucosa: An experimental study in the rat. *J Oral Pathol* 1983;12:187–198.

Raque CJ, Biondo RV, Keeran MG, et al. Snuff dippers keratosis (snuff-induced leukoplakia). *South Med J* 1975;68: 565–568.

Smith JF. Snuff-dippers lesions. A ten-year follow-up. *Arch Otolaryngol* 1975;101:276–277.

Summerlin DJ, Dunipace A, Potter R. Histologic effects of smokeless tobacco and alcohol on the pouch mucosa and organs of the Syrian hamster. *J Oral Pathol Med* 1992;21:105–108.

Taybos G. Oral changes associated with tobacco use. *Am J Med Sci* 2003;326:179–182.

Smoker's Melanosis

■ Definition

Smoker's melanosis is a benign focal pigmentation of the oral mucosa more commonly encountered in women after the third decade of life.

■ Etiology

The lesion is thought to represent an increase in the melanin production in the basal cell layer of the epithelium stimulated by tobacco.

■ Main Clinical Features

- Multiple brown pigmented macules or plaques localized mainly in the anterior mandibular attached gingiva and interdental papillae
- The buccal mucosa and palate are less commonly affected by melanosis induced by smoking

■ Diagnosis

The diagnosis is based on the history and the clinical features.

■ Differential Diagnosis

- Racial melanosis
- Amalgam tattoo
- Traumatic melanosis
- Pigmented nevi
- Drug-induced melanosis
- Lentigo melanotic macule
- Addison disease
- Peutz–Jeghers syndrome
- Albright syndrome
- Von Recklinghausen disease

■ Treatment

Basic Guidelines

- No treatment is required.
- The lesions gradually diminish after smoking cessation and may disappear after a period of a few months or years.

Suggested Therapies

Smoking cessation.

References

Axell T, Hedin CA. Epidemiologic study of excessive oral melanin pigmentation with special reference to the influence of tobacco habits. *Scand J Dent Res* 1982;90: 434–442.

Hedin CA. Smoker's melanosis. Occurrence and localization in the attached gingiva. *Arch Dermatol* 1977;113: 1533–1538.

Hedin CA, Axell T. Oral melanin pigmentation in 467 Thai and Malaysian people with special emphasis on smoker's melanosis. *J Oral Pathol Med* 1991;20:8–12.

Hedin C, Pindborg JJ, Daftary DK, Mehta FS. Melanin depigmentation of the palatal mucosa in reverse smokers: A preliminary study. *J Oral Pathol Med* 1992;21:440–444.

Hedin CA, Pindborg JJ, Axel T. Disappearance of smoker's melanosis after reducing smoking. *J Oral Pathol Med* 1993;22:228–230.

Squamous Cell Carcinoma

■ Definition

Oral squamous cell carcinoma is by far the most common malignant neoplasm. It accounts for more than 90% of all oral malignancies.

■ Etiology

The etiology is unknown. However, several predisposing factors have been implicated. The most important are tobacco use, alcohol consumption, human papillomavirus (types 16, 18, and 33) and chronic sun exposure (for lip carcinoma only).

■ Main Clinical Features

Clinically, oral squamous cell carcinoma has a broad spectrum of features and may mimic a variety of diseases.

Early Stage

- Asymptomatic red or white plaque or both
- Erosion or superficial small ulcer
- Small exophytic mass
- Erosion with crust formation, as in lip carcinoma

Advanced Stage

- Painful deep ulcer with irregular vegetating surface, elevated border, and hard base
- Large exophytic mass with or without ulceration
- Infiltrating hardness of the oral tissues
- Periodontal destruction and tooth mobility
- Regional lymph nodes enlargement
- Longstanding indurated lesions are always suspect for malignancy
- The posterior lateral border and the ventral surface of the tongue, the floor of the mouth, and the gingiva are the most commonly affected sites
- The prognosis depends on the stage at diagnosis and the histologic pattern

■ Diagnosis

The clinical diagnosis should be confirmed by a biopsy and histopathologic examination.

■ Differential Diagnosis

- Traumatic ulcer
- Aphthous ulcer
- Tuberculous ulcer
- Syphilitic ulcer
- Eosinophilic ulcer
- Leukoplakia
- Erythroplakia
- Pyogenic granuloma
- Necrotizing sialadenometaplasia
- Wegener granulomatosis
- Malignant granuloma
- Non-Hodgkin lymphoma
- Benign and malignant tumors of minor salivary glands

■ Treatment

Basic Guidelines

- The diagnosis must be made as soon as possible and treatment initiated promptly.
- The prognosis depends mainly on the clinical stage at diagnosis and the choice of treatment modalities.
- Before treatment decision, close collaboration between the stomatologist, radiologist, and oncologist is necessary.
- After treatment a follow-up program is important as the risk for recurrence is relatively high.
- Cessation of smoking and alcohol is essential.

Suggested Therapies

Treatment of oral squamous cell carcinoma consists of surgical excision, radiation therapy, or combination of both. Chemotherapy is also been used in combination with surgery and radiation. The decision for monotherapy or combination of therapies depend on the clinical stage of the disease, and the age and general health of the patient.

Surgical Treatment

The main aim of surgical treatment is total excision of the tumor with a wide 1.5–2.5 cm margin of surrounding healthy tissues in all three dimensions.

In cases of bony involvement a peripheral, partial and finally hemi-mandibulectomy or hemi-maxillectomy should be performed.

Several surgical methods allow complete removal and immediate reconstruction of the missing soft and hard tissues to achieve a better functional and cosmetic result for the patient. According to the nature of the defect, skin or bony grafts are used for reconstructive purposes as well as the several types of cutaneous, myocutaneous, or osseomyocutaneous flaps. These flaps can be either local or regional or can be applied as free microvascular flaps from the iliac crest, fibula, radius, and scapula as well as the serratus and latissimus dorsi muscles.

Besides elimination of the primary site of the tumor, surgical management includes several types of surgical neck dissections to remove all possible regional lymph node metastases.

Despite recent improvement in surgical techniques and diagnostic tools, the overall postoperative 5-year survival rate of squamous cell carcinoma is still poor. Consequently, prevention and early diagnosis of oral squamous cell carcinoma is of great importance.

Radiotherapy

Modern era radiotherapy plays an important role in the radical treatment of patients with oral squamous cell carcinomas and has improved local control and their quality of life. It can be combined with surgery, pre- or postoperatively, and/or chemotherapy or can be used as the sole method of curative treatment. Radiotherapy combined with chemotherapy has the extra advantage of organ preservation. The introduction of multileaf linear accelerators and new software making use of computerized tomography (CT), magnetic resonance (MR), and, recently, positron emission tomography (PET) images, resulted in the development of three-dimensional conformal radiotherapy (3DCRT) and, even most recently, in what is called intensity modulated radiotherapy (IMRT).

Radiotherapy has been used in combination with chemotherapy in nonresectable oral squamous cell carcinoma in preparation for surgery, or the two together in organ preserving, radical curative attempts. A meta-analysis published in 2003 concluded that cisplatin, carboplatin, mitomycin-C and 5-fluorouracil (FU) single drug or combinations of 5-FU with one of other drugs, combined with simultaneous radiotherapy leads to a profound survival benefit in unresectable head and neck cancer patients irrespective of the fractionation schedule.

Radiotherapy can also be used as brachytherapy with interstitial radioactive isotopes, either in the form of temporary implants of radioactive iridium or after loading machines, thus achieving excellent conformity of radiation dose to the gross tumor volume.

Hyperthermia is another type of treatment that can be combined with radiotherapy with additive cancer killing effect and nonadditive side effects.

While modern era radiotherapy in combination with other modalities has improved life expectancy and organ preservation of patients with oral cavity squamous cell carcinomas, prophylactic reduction of alcohol and cigarette consumption is the best way to reduce morbidity and mortality.

Chemotherapy

Chemotherapy was used in the past in advanced disease or for recurrence after surgery and/or radiotherapy. During the last few years chemotherapy has been used more in a better and effective way. The term induction chemotherapy has gained ground and several investigators have studied ways to improve the final outcome of the disease. To be able to start treatment with chemotherapy before any radiation or surgery produced hope and has shown a higher efficacy and response rate of the tumors to the cytotoxic agents.

Chemotherapy was initiated in the treatment of head and neck cancers, including the oral carcinomas, by the introduction of the cytotoxic drug cisplatin. Cisplatin in combination with other agents started producing reasonably effective results in advanced stage. Cisplatin combined with 5-FU is one of the most effective combination and one of the standard treatments. Other cytotoxic agents that have been used in combinations are methotrexate, bleomycin, hydroxyurea, and vinca alkaloids. Taxanes, e.g., paclitaxel combined with a cisplatin analogue carboplatin, has also been shown to be highly effective and can be considered a first-line treatment. Response rates of 24–39% in advanced disease have been recorded. Chemotherapy for recurrent or advanced metastatic disease may not produce sufficient cure rates but there is a degree of response and prolongation of survival.

Two other chemotherapeutical strategies have been used over the past 10 years to improve the treatment efficacy on the whole: a) chemotherapy before any other treatment (induction chemotherapy) and b) combination of chemotherapy with radiotherapy (concurrent treatment). The rationale behind induction chemotherapy is based on better drug delivery to the tumor when the vascular bed is intact, and the possible eradication of micrometastatic disease. The last may allow the drug dose to be more efficient and thus improve compliance. Response can result in less extensive surgery or tumors possibly become operable. The response rate of patients after induction chemotherapy has been highly increased. Concurrent treatment is gaining ground.

References

Al-Sarraf M, Pajak TF, Byhardt RW, et al. Postoperative radiotherapy with concurrent cisplatin appears to improve locoregional control of advanced, resectable bend and neck cancer. *Int J Radiat Oncol Biol Phys* 1997;37: 777–782.

Bernier J, Domenge C, Eschwege F. Chemo-radiotherapy, as compared to radiotherapy alone, significantly increases disease-free and overall survival in head and neck cancer patients after surgery: Results of EORTC phase III trial 22931 [abstract]. *Int J Radiat Oncol Phys* 2001;51 (suppl 1):1.

Budach W, Hehr T, Beika C, Dietz K. Radiotherapy combined with cisplatin/carboplatin, mitomycin C and 5FU, single drug or two drug chemotherapy compared to radiotherapy alone in unresectable head and neck cancer: A meta analysis [abstract]. No. 684, *Eur J Cancer* 2003; 1(suppl):5206.

Cawson RA, Binnie WH, Barrett AW, Wright JM. *Lucas's Pathology of Tumors of the Oral Tissues*, 5th edition. Churchill Livingstone: London, 1998.

Cooper JS, Pajak TF, Forastiere AA. Postoperative concurrent radiochemotherapy in high-risk SCCA of the head and neck [abstract]. *J Clin Oncol* 2002;21:226A.

Dische S, Saunders M, Barret A, et al. A randomized multicenter trial of CHART versus conventional radiotherapy in head end neck cancer. *Radiother Oncol* 1997;44:123–136.

Horiot J-C, Bontemps P, van den Bogaert W. Accelerated fractionation compared to conventional fractionation improved loco regional control in the radiotherapy of advanced head and neck cancers: results of the EORTC 22851 trial. *Radiother Oncol* 1997;44:111–121.

Mendenhall WM, Stringer SP, Moore GJ, et al. Squamous cell carcinoma of the base of tongue treated with external-beam radiation therapy: A preferred alternative to surgery. *Int J Radiat Oncol Biol Phys* 1999;45(suppl):197.

Sciubba JJ. Oral cancer. The importance of early diagnosis and treatment. *Am J Clin Dermatol* 2001;2:239–251.

Shah JP. *Head and Neck Surgery*, Wolfe Medical Publications: Hong Kong, 1990.

Stathopoulos GP, Rigatos S, Papakostas P, Fountzilas G. Effectiveness of paclitaxel and carboplatin combination in heavily pretreated patients with head and neck cancers. *Eur J Cancer* 1997;33:1780–1783.

Vokes EE, Weichselbaum RR, Lippman SM, Kikong W. Head and neck medical progress. *N Engl J Med* 1993;328:184–194.

Streptococcal Gingivostomatitis

▨ Definition

Streptococcal gingivostomatitis is a debatable infectious oral disease.

▨ Etiology

The main cause is group A β-hemolytic streptococci and rarely other strains.

▨ Main Clinical Features

- Redness and edema
- Superficial erosions covered with a whitish smear
- The lesions are usually localized on the gingiva, rarely in other oral regions
- Mild fever
- Malaise
- Submandibular lymphadenopathy

▨ Diagnosis

The diagnosis should be confirmed by Gram staining and culture.

▨ Differential Diagnosis

- Herpetic gingivostomatitis
- Necrotizing ulcerative gingivitis
- Staphylococcal infection
- Trauma

▨ Treatment

Basic Guidelines

- Laboratory identification of streptococci is important before treatment.
- Early diagnosis and treatment is important.

Suggested Therapies

Systemic Treatment

- Oral penicillin V 500–750 mg/day for 6–8 days is recommended.
- Oral cephalosporins such as cefaclor 250–500 mg every 8 hours or cephalexin 250–500 mg every 8 hours for 4–6 days may also be used.
- Macrolides such as erythromycin 250–500 mg every 8 hours or clarithromycin 250–500 mg twice daily for 4–6 days may be used as a second-line treatment.

Topical Treatment

0.2 % chlorhexidine gluconate may be used as mouthwash 3–4 times daily.

References

Brook I. Antibacterial therapy for acute group a streptococcal pharyngotonsillitis: Short-course versus traditional 10-day or regimens. *Paediatr Drugs* 2002;4:747–754.

Katz J, Guelmann M, Rudolph M, Ruskin J. Acute streptococcal infection of the gingiva, lower lip and pharynx: A case report. *J Periodontol* 2002;73:1392–1395.

Kuriyama T, Karasawa T, Kanagawa K, et al. Antimicrobial susceptibility of major pathogens of orofacial odontogenic infections to 11 beta-lactam antibiotics. *Oral Microbiol Immunol* 2002;17:285–289.

Laskaris G. *Color Atlas of Oral Diseases*, 3rd edition. Thieme Verlag: Stuttgart, 2003.

Sweet Syndrome

■ Definition

Sweet syndrome or acute febrile neutrophilic dermatosis is an uncommon acute neutrophilic dermatosis associated with systemic manifestations.

■ Etiology

The etiology is unknown. However, the frequent association with infections, autoimmune diseases, inflammatory bowel disease, lymphocytic malignancies, and drugs suggest a hypersensitivity reaction.

■ Classification

On the basis of underlying etiology the syndrome is subdivided into five types: a) idiopathic, b) drug-induced, c) malignancy-associated, d) bowel disease–associated, and e) pregnancy-associated.

■ Main Clinical Features

Skin and systemic manifestations are the main clinical features of Sweet syndrome. The oral mucosa is rarely affected.

Oral Lesions

Erythema and painful aphthous-like lesions of varying size are the most common oral lesions. The lip, tongue, buccal mucosa, and palate are more frequently affected

Skin Lesions

Nonpruritic, multiple, edematous and erythematous papules and plaques are the most common lesions. Vesiculobullous lesions that rupture leading to ulcerations may also occur. The head, neck and the dorsal aspect of the hands are more frequently affected

Systemic Manifestations

Fever (38–39 °C), leukocytosis, arthralgias, arthritis, myalgias, and ocular involvement are the most common manifestations. Renal, liver, respiratory and pancreas are rarely involved

■ Diagnosis

The diagnosis is mainly based on clinical criteria. Biopsy and histopathologic examination of skin lesions and leukocytosis with neutrophilia are very helpful.

■ Differential Diagnosis

- Aphthous ulcer
- Behçet disease
- FAPA syndrome
- Erythema multiforme
- Wegener granulomatosis
- Pyoderma gangrenosum
- Pyostomatitis vegetans
- Sarcoidosis
- Lupus erythematosus
- Other neutrophilic dermatosis
- Systemic mycoses
- Leishmaniasis
- Non-Hodgkin lymphoma

■ Treatment

Basic Guidelines

- The oral lesions are unusual and part of the systemic disease.
- Treatment of oral lesions should be part of the systemic treatment.
- Clinicians must bear in mind the possibility of association with an underlying disorder including malignancy.
- The systemic treatment of the disease must be provided by a specialist.

Suggested Therapies

Systemic Treatment

- Corticosteroids are the drugs of choice for the treatment of Sweet syndrome. Prednisone

0.5–1 mg/kg per day for 3–6 weeks is usually enough to control the disease. In resistant cases, low-dose prednisone, 20–30 mg/day for an additional 1–3 months may be necessary to prevent recurrence. When the disease is associated with a recognized infection (e.g., *Streptococcus, Staphylococcus*) antibiotics may be helpful.

- Dapsone 100–200 mg/day, or colchicine 1–2 mg/day, or potassium iodine 900 mg/day are the main alternative drugs.
- Nonsteroidal anti-inflammatory drugs, thalidomide, cyclosporine, tacrolimus and interferon alpha have been reported to be useful.

Topical Treatment

Topical treatment of oral lesions is necessary to reduce the pain and the duration of the ulcers. Triamcinolone acetonide in Orabase or 0.05% clobetasol propionate gel is applied to the ulcer three to six times a day for 1–2 weeks. Amlexanox 5% oral paste and topical anesthetics such as 2% viscous lidocaine may improve the symptoms. Intralesional injection of corticosteroids may be helpful. Topical super potent or intralesional corticosteroids can result in an improvement of localized cutaneous lesions.

References

Bayer-Garner IB, Cottler-Fox M, Smoller BR. Sweet syndrome in multiple myeloma: A series of six cases. *J Cutan Pathol* 2003;30:261–264.

Fellermann K, Rudolph B, Witthoft T, et al. Sweet's syndrome and erythema nodosum in ulcerative colitis, refractory to steroids: Successful treatment with tacrolimus. *Med Klin* 2001;96:105–108.

Femiano F, Gombos F, Scully C. Sweet's syndrome: Recurrent oral ulceration, pyrexia, thrombophlebitis and cutaneous lesions. *Oral Surg Oral Med Oral Pathol Oral Radiol Endod* 2003;95:324–327.

Khan-Durani B, Jappe U. Drug-induced Sweet's syndrome in acne causes by different tetracycline: Case report and review of the literatue. *Br J Dermatol* 2002;147:558–562.

Notani K,Kobayashi S, Kondoh K, et al. A case of Sweet's syndrome (acute febrile neutrophilic dermatosis) with palatal ulceration. *Oral Surg Oral Med Oral Pathol Oral Radiol Endod* 2000;89:477–479.

Su WPD, Liu HNH. Diagnostic criteria for Sweet's syndrome. *Cutis* 1986;37:167–174.

Syphilis

Definition

Syphilis is a sexually transmitted infectious disease involving several organs and systems.

Etiology

The causative organism is *Treponema pallidum.*

Classification

- Congenital
- Acquired (primary, secondary, tertiary)

Main Clinical Features

Approximately 5–10% of primary and over 40% of secondary syphilis manifests in the oral mucosa. Tertiary syphilis is now extremely rare. The main clinical manifestations of acquired syphilis are mucocutaneous lesions and constitutional signs and symptoms.

Oral Lesions

- Primary syphilis presents as an ulcer (chancre), always associated with regional lymph node enlargement. The tongue, palate, and lips are most commonly affected
- Secondary syphilis usually presents as mucous patches and rarely as macular syphilides (roseola), papular syphilides, and condylomata lata
- Tertiary syphilis presents as gumma, atrophic glossitis, and interstitial glossitis

Genital Lesions

- Primary syphilitic ulcer
- Mucous patches of secondary syphilis

Skin Lesions

- Secondary syphilis: characterized by several skin signs and lesions such as pruritus, macules, papules, nodules, pustules, and follicular and nails lesions. Condylomata lata may appear in moist skin areas, particularly in the perigenital and perianal areas.

- Tertiary syphilis: classic lesion is the gumma, which occurs mainly on the legs, scalp, face, and chest.

Constitutional Signs and Symptoms

- Headache
- Malaise
- Low-grade fever
- Lacrimation
- Sore throat
- Appetite loss
- Weight loss
- Polyarthralgia
- Myalgias
- Splenomegaly
- Generalized lymphadenopathy

Diagnosis

The clinical diagnosis should be confirmed by dark-field microscopic examination and serologic tests (Venereal Diseases Research Laboratories [VDRL], rapid plasma reagin [RPR], fluorescent treponemal antibody-absorption [FTA-ABS], *Treponema pallidum* immobilization [TPI], *Treponema pallidum* hemagglutination [TPHA], solid phase hemadsorption test [SPHA]).

Differential Diagnosis

- Traumatic ulcer
- Aphthous ulcer
- Behçet disease
- Herpes simplex
- Cinnamon contact stomatitis
- Infectious mononucleosis
- Chancroid
- Tuberculosis
- Candidiasis
- Erythema multiforme
- Lichen planus
- Leukoplakia
- Lupus erythematosus
- Wegener granulomatosis
- Squamous cell carcinoma

▩ Treatment

Basic Guidelines

- Intramuscular penicillin is still the mainstay of treatment for all stages of syphilis.
- The dose of penicillin depends on the stage of the disease.
- Treatment of oral syphilis must be subjected to the rules that guide the treatment of syphilis treatment.
- No topical treatment is necessary.
- The treatment of oral syphilis must be provided by a specialist.
- Follow-up serologic tests (VDRL, TPHA) are recommended periodically (1, 3, and 6 months) after treatment of early syphilis and later every 6 months for 3–6 years.

Suggested Therapies

- Benzathine penicillin in a single i.m. dose of 2.4 MU is recommended for primary and secondary syphilis as well as in early latent syphilis (<1 year in duration). For latent syphilis (>1 year in duration) benzathine penicillin in an i.m. dose of 2.4 MU weekly for 3 weeks is recommended.

- Procaine penicillin in an i.m. dose of 600–1200 mg/day over 10–12 continuous days for early syphilis and over 18–22 days for late latent syphilis may be used as an alternative regimen. Probenecid 10 mg twice daily together with procaine penicillin is recommended for better results.
- Alternative regimens for penicillin-allergic patients are: erythromycin 500 mg four times daily for 2 weeks or tetracycline 500 mg for times daily for 2 weeks or doxycycline 200 mg daily for 2 weeks in early syphilis and the same dose for 4 weeks in late latent syphilis.

References

Gohl T, Van Voorst Vlader PC. European guidelines for the management of syphilis. *Int J STD AIDS* 2001;12(suppl 3):14–26.

Laskaris G. *Color Atlas of Oral Diseases*, 3rd edition, pp. 186–93. Thieme Verlag: Stuttgart, 2003.

Van Voorst Vlader PC. Syphilis management and treatment. *Dermatol Clin* 1998;16: 699–711.

Waugh MA. Syphilis. In: Katsambas AD, Lotti TM (editors). *European Handbook of Dermatological Treatments*, 2nd edition, pp. 512–518. Springer-Verlag: Berlin, 2003.

World Health Organization. Management of sexually transmitted diseases. Geneva, WHO, 2001.

Thermal Burn

■ Definition

Thermal burn is a common mucosal lesion.

■ Etiology

The burn is caused by contact with extremely hot food, liquids, or objects.

■ Main Clinical Features

- Red painful lesion that may desquamate and be covered by a white pseudomembrane
- The most commonly affected areas are the palate, buccal mucosa, lips, and tongue

■ Diagnosis

The diagnosis is based on the history and clinical features.

■ Differential Diagnosis

- Chemical burns
- Traumatic ulcers
- Herpes simplex
- Vesiculobullous disease
- Stomatitis medicamentosa
- Cinnamon contact stomatitis

■ Treatment

Basic Guidelines

- Avoid spices, hot and hard foods.
- It is important to examine whether there are any other lesions present in the oral cavity as thermal burn is usually a solitary lesion.

Suggested Therapies

- The lesion usually heals within a week with no additional treatment. If the pain is intense, a topical anesthetic (dyclonine hydrochloride) may be applied, although the relief provided is of short duration.
- Cold chamomile mouthwashes are helpful.

References

Chadwick RG. The thermal insulating effects of five dental gloves. *J Oral Rehabil* 2000;27:341–343.

Cullen R. The oral burn syndrome and its effects on dental implants. *J Oral Implantol* 1998;24:219–221.

Hashem FK, Al Khayal Z. Oral burn contractures in children. *Ann Plast Surg* 2003;51:468–471.

Milano M. Oral electrical and thermal burns in children: Review and report of case. *J Dent Child* 1999;66:116–119.

Speyer M, Joe J, Davidson JM, et al. Thermal injury patterns and tensile strength of canine oral mucosa after carbon dioxide laser incisions. *Laryngoscope* 1996;106:845–850.

Toxic Epidermal Necrolysis

■ Definition

Toxic epidermal necrolysis or Lyell disease is an acute, life-threatening clinicopathologic entity characterized by extensive detachment of full-thickness epidermis and mucous membranes.

■ Etiology

Usually drugs are responsible, but other factors (viruses, bacteria, AIDS, systemic diseases) may also be involved in rare cases.

■ Main Clinical Features

The disease usually begins with fever, cough, sore throat, and burning eyes, preceding by 1–3 days the skin and mucous membrane lesions. Mucous membrane involvement is present in 85–95 % of cases.

Oral Mucosa

The oral lesions appear as diffuse erythema, blistering and painful, widespread erosions. Increased salivation is common

Other Mucosae

Several other mucosae are usually affected (eyes, pharynx, esophagus, genitalia, anus). The gastrointestinal and respiratory tracts may be involved

Skin

The skin lesions manifest as sheet-like loss of epidermis raised by flaccid blisters. Detachment of the full thickness of the epidermis over pressure areas leaves a dark-red oozing dermis. The entire skin surface may be involved, with up to 100 % of the epidermis sloughing off. Nikolsky sign is positive

■ Diagnosis

The diagnosis is usually made clinically. However, histopathologic examination should confirm the diagnosis.

■ Differential Diagnosis

- Erythema multiforme, major
- Staphylococcal scalded skin syndrome
- Pemphigus vulgaris
- Paraneoplastic pemphigus

■ Treatment

Basic Guidelines

- Management of patients must be undertaken as soon as possible in intensive care units or in burn units.
- Medical transport requires particular attention to the skin.
- Palliative treatment of oral lesions is necessary.
- Ocular lesions require daily examination by an ophthalmologist.
- Generally, therapy of this self-limiting disease relies on symptomatic management.
- The details of the treatment are beyond the scope of this book.

Suggested Therapies

- Symptomatic.
- The role of systemic corticosteroids is controversial.
- Cyclosporine and cyclophosphamide are alternative drugs.
- Plasmapheresis is occasionally helpful.
- Oral debris should be removed and antiseptic mouthwashes used several times each day.
- Surgical care and rehabilitation are sometimes necessary.

References

Paquet P, Pierard GE. Erythema multiforme and toxic epidermal necrolysis: A comparative study. *Am J Dermatopathol* 1997;19:127–132.
Roujeau J-C. Drug-induced toxic epidermal necrolysis. II. Current aspects. *Clin Dermatol* 1993;11:493–500.
Smoot III EC. Treatment issues in the care of patients with toxic epidermal necrolysis. *Burns* 1999;25:439–442.
Viard I, Wehrli P, Bullani R, et al. Inhibition of toxic epidermal necrolysis by blockade of CD95 with human intravenous immunoglobulin. *Science* 1998;282:490–492.

Traumatic Ulcer

■ Definition

Traumatic ulcer is one of the most common mucosal lesions in oral medicine.

■ Etiology

Mechanical damage from sharp or broken teeth, rough fillings, denture irritation, sharp foreign bodies, biting of the mucosa, and dental instruments are the most common causes.

■ Main Clinical Features

- Usually it appears as a single painful ulcer with a smooth red or white-yellow surface and red halo
- The ulcer is usually soft on palpation
- When the trauma is intense and chronic the ulcer can have a vegetating surface and indurated borders mimicking a carcinoma
- The size of the ulcer varies from a few millimeters to several centimeters
- Lateral margins of the tongue, buccal mucosa, lips, buccoalveolar grooves, palate, and floor of the mouth are the sites of predilection

■ Diagnosis

The diagnosis is usually based on the history and the clinical examination. However, occasionally a biopsy is necessary to rule out malignancy.

■ Differential Diagnosis

- Squamous cell carcinoma
- Aphthous ulcer
- Chemical burn
- Thermal burn
- Eosinophilic ulcer
- Syphilitic ulcer
- Tuberculous ulcer
- Drug-induced ulceration

■ Treatment

Basic Guidelines

- Removal of any obvious cause of injury.
- Reexamine the patient 7–10 days after the removal of the probable traumatic cause.
- If the lesion persists after 2 weeks, take a biopsy.

Suggested Therapies

- Removal or correction of the traumatic cause usually leads to rapid healing of the ulcer.
- Topical rinses with hydrogen peroxide or carbamide peroxide promote faster healing.
- Topical corticosteroid ointments or gel improve the symptoms and help healing.
- Systemic oral corticosteroids in low doses and for a short time, e.g., prednisone 15–20 mg for 4–6 days, can be used successfully for chronic and painful traumatic ulcers only.

References

Gaffar A. Recurrent oral ulcers: An overview. *Compend Contin Educ Dent Suppl* 2001;32:4–6.

Garcia-Pola Vallejo MJ, Martinez Diaz-Canel AI, Garcia Martin JM, Gonzalez Garcia M. Risk factors for oral soft tissue lesions in an adult Spanish population. *Comm Dent Oral Epidemiol* 2002;30:277–285.

Jainkittivong A, Aneksuk V, Langlais RP. Oral mucosal conditions in elderly dental patients. *Oral Dis* 2002;8:218–223.

Laskaris G. *Color Atlas of Oral Diseases*, 3rd edition. Thieme Verlag: Stuttgart, 2003.

Slayton RL. Treatment alternatives for sublingual traumatic ulceration (Riga-Fede disease). *Pediatr Dent* 2000;22:413–414.

Trigeminal Neuralgia (Idiopathic)

◼ Definition

Idiopathic trigeminal neuralgia or tic douloureux is a relatively common condition characterized by recurrent unilateral episodes of sharp paroxysms of pain.

◼ Etiology

The etiology of trigeminal neuralgia is unknown.

◼ Main Clinical Features

- Pain is confined along one or more divisions of the trigeminal nerve
- Paroxysmal pain attacks last between a few seconds and 2–3 minutes
- Pain is sudden, sharp, intense, stabbing, or burning, and usually develops in the oral cavity, shooting toward the eye, ear, and nostril
- Pain may be triggered or precipitated by eating, touching, washing the face, and brushing the teeth
- Characteristically patients hold the face during the attack, even while talking
- Paroxysms of pain became progressively more frequent and the remissions shorter
- Spontaneous remissions may last for several months or years
- Neurologic examination is usually normal, except in rare cases where trigeminal neuralgia is a symptom of multiple sclerosis or a brain malignancy

◼ Diagnosis

The diagnosis is based on the clinical features.

◼ Differential Diagnosis

- Trigeminal neuralgia (symptomatic)
- Glossopharyngeal neuralgia
- Nervus intermedius neuralgia
- Superior laryngeal nerve neuralgia
- Central causes of facial pain
- Multiple sclerosis
- Other causes of facial pain

◼ Treatment

Basic Guidelines

- Before treatment a neurologic examination is necessary to rule out other causes of facial pain or neurologic diseases.
- A careful oral examination should be done to remove probable local triggering foci (e.g., gingivitis, periodontitis, carries, pulpitis).
- Noninvasive treatment should be attempted before any invasive procedures.
- There is no curative treatment as relapse is common.
- The treatment of idiopathic trigeminal neuralgia must be provided by a specialist.

Suggested Therapies

Drug Therapies

- Carbamazepine 400–1000 mg/day is the first-line drug. It usually controls the pain. However, recurrences are common and the drug has numerous side effects (depressive action on hematopoiesis, nausea, drowsiness).
- Gabapentin is also a first-line drug for the treatment of idiopathic trigeminal neuralgia. The initial dose is usually 600 mg/day, which may be gradually increased to 900–1200 mg/day. This drug has fewer side effects than carbamazepine.
- Diazepam 2–5 mg three times daily in combination with oral prednisone 10–15 mg/day usually gives excellent results in my experience. The dose of prednisone, when the pain is controlled, may be reduced to 5 mg/day and later stopped.
- Alternatively, clonazepam, baclofen and other agents have been used either alone or in combination. The response to these drugs is unpredictable.

Nondrug Therapies

Several nondrug therapies have been recommended if pharmacologic treatment is unsuccessful. The efficacy of these procedures is moderate to little. The most popular of nondrug therapies are: transcutaneous electrical nerve stimulation, lasers, and several surgical approaches that may vary in invasiveness and effect (e. g., microvascular decompression, percutaneous trigeminal ganglion compression, radiosurgery etc). Alcohol injection of the trigeminal ganglion and rhizotomy have also been used.

References

Cheshire WP. Defining the role of gabapentin in the treatment of trigeminal neuralgia: a retrospective study. *J Pain* 2002;3:137–142.

Fisher A, Zakrzewska JM, Patsalos PN. Trigeminal neuralgia: Current treatments and future developments. *Expert Opin Emerg Drugs* 2003;8:123–143.

Goss BW, Frighetto L, DeSalles AA, et al. Linear accelerator radiosurgery using 90 gray for essential trigeminal neuralgia: Results and dose volume histogram analysis. *Neurosurgery* 2003;53:823–828.

Hitotsumatsu T, Matsushima T, Inoue T. Microvasular decompression for treatment of trigeminal neuralgia, hemifacial spasm and glossopharyngeal neuralgia: Three surgical approach variations [technical note]. *Neurosurgery* 2003;53:1436–1441.

Mangini F. *Headache and Facial Pain.* Thieme Verlag: Stuttgart, 1999.

Petit JH, Heman JM, Nagda S, et al. Radiosurgical treatment of trigeminal neuralgia: Evaluating quality of life and treatment outcome. *Int J Radiat Oncol Biol Phys* 2003;56: 1147–1153.

Tuberculosis

Definition

Tuberculosis is a chronic granulomatous infectious disease.

Etiology

The causative organism is *Mycobacterium tuberculosis.*

Main Clinical Features

Oral lesions of tuberculosis usually represent secondary infection from the primary pulmonary lesions. The prevalence of the oral lesions varies from 0.5% to 1.5%. Rarely, oral lesions may be the only manifestation of otherwise silent tuberculosis.

Oral Tuberculosis

- Irregular ulcer with a thin border is the most common feature. The surrounding tissues are slightly indurated with inflammation
- Nodular or granular lesions may also occur
- Tongue, palate, buccal mucosa, gingiva, and lips are more frequently affected
- Regional lymphadenopathy usually accompanies the oral lesions
- Tuberculous osteomyelitis of the jaws may rarely occur

Pulmonary Tuberculosis

- Low-grade fever
- Anorexia and malaise
- Cough and night sweats
- Weight loss
- Chest pain
- Hemoptysis
- Generalized lymphadenopathy

Diagnosis

A clinical suspicion of oral tuberculosis should be confirmed by a biopsy and histopathologic examination, mycobacterial examination of the sputum culture. Chest radiography and Mantoux tuberculin skin test are also done.

Differential Diagnosis

- Traumatic ulcer
- Aphthous ulcer
- Pyostomatitis vegetans
- Eosinophilic ulcer
- Syphilis
- Sarcoidosis
- Systemic mycoses
- Wegener granulomatosis
- Malignant granuloma
- Non-Hodgkin lymphoma
- Squamous cell carcinoma

Treatment

Basic Guidelines

- Clinical evaluation: Poor general condition, miliary or central nervous system disease, renal and liver dysfunction, current medications for untreated diseases, psychiatric or other evidence for expected poor compliance.
- Epidemiologic evaluation: Exposure to persons with prolonged positive cultures or known drug resistance and travel to areas with endemic drug resistance denote probable resistant disease.
- Radiographic evaluation: Cavitary or miliary disease requires prolonged treatment.
- Microscopic examination and culture and sensitivity for acid-fast bacilli.
- Purified protein derivative (PPD)-tuberculin skin test: A negative test does not exclude active disease.
- Complete blood count, platelet count, serum glutamic-oxaloacetic transaminase [SGOT], serum glutamic-pyruvic transaminase [SGPT], bilirubin, alkaline phosphatase, serum creatinine, urinalysis.
- Testing of visual acuity and red-green influenced by the local availability of imaging, culture, and susceptibility of testing facilities. Use of second-line drugs requires previous experience or consultation with an expert physician.
- The treatment of oral tuberculosis must be provided by a specialist.

Suggested Therapies

Treatment Regimen For the Initial 2-Month Phase

Adults with previously untreated tuberculosis are typically given four medications for 2 months: a) isoniazid (INH, 5 mg/kg up to 300 mg/day), b) rifampin (10 mg/kg up to 600 mg/day), c) pyrazinamide (40–55 kg body-weight, 1000 mg/day; 56–75 kg bodyweight, 1500 mg/day; 76–90 kg bodyweight 2000 mg/day; it may be withheld in severe liver disease, gout, and pregnancy), and d) ethambutol (40–55 kg, 800 mg/day; 56–75 kg, 1200 mg/day; 76–90 kg, 1600 mg/day).

Treatment Regimen After the Initial 2-Month Phase

Continuation phase lasts 4–7 months, typically with isoniazid and rifampin. Extended treatment is recommended for patients with drug-susceptible pulmonary tuberculosis who have cavitation noted on the initial chest film and who have positive sputum cultures after 2 months of treatment or if the initial phase of treatment did not include pyrazinamide.

Monitoring for Disease Improvement and Adverse Drug Reactions During Treatment

- Monthly clinical evaluation to monitor the course of oral and lung lesions, identify possible adverse effects of the antituberculosis medications, and assess adherence.
- Monthly sputum specimen for microscopic examination and culture until two consecutive specimens are negative on culture.
- Monthly radiologic and blood tests initially and thereafter according to the course of the disease.

References

Cakan A, Mutlu Z, Ozsoz A, et al. Tuberculosis of oral mucosa. *Monaldi Arch Chest Dis* 2001;58:315–317.

Joint Statement on Treatment of Tuberculosis of the American Thoracic Society, CDC, and the Infectious Diseases Society of America. *Am J Resp Crit Care Med* 2003;187: 603–662.

Nagabhushana D, Balaji RB, Rajeshwari A, Mamatha GP. Oral tuberculosis: A case report. *J Indian Soc Pedod Prev Dent* 2003;21;16–18.

Sierra C, Fortun J, Barros C, et al. Extra-laryngeal head and neck tuberculosis. *Clin Microbiol Infect* 2000;6:644–648.

Uremic Stomatitis

■ Definition

Uremic stomatitis is a rare complication that may occur in patients with acute or chronic renal failure.

■ Etiology

The etiology is unknown. A pathogenetic hypothesis is that stomatitis may be a reaction of the oral mucosa to toxins or to the action of ammonia, or that urease produced by the oral microflora may degrade urea secreted in saliva.

■ Main Clinical Features

- Painful superficial ulcerations, covered by necrotic pseudomembranes
- Painful diffuse edematous erythema covered by a thick grayish pseudomembrane
- Local hemorrhage and ecchymoses
- Multiple painful hyperkeratotic plaques
- Xerostomia, burning sensation, uriniferous breath odor, unpleasant taste, candidiasis, viral and bacterial infections

■ Diagnosis

The diagnosis is supported by the history, urinalysis and blood urea level.

■ Differential Diagnosis

- Candidiasis
- Cinnamon contact stomatitis
- Hairy leukoplakia
- Drug reactions
- Allergic stomatitis
- Necrotizing ulcerative stomatitis
- Agranulocytosis
- Aplastic anemia

■ Treatment

Basic Guidelines

- A full medical history is essential for final diagnosis before treatment.
- The oral clinician should collaborate with the specialist nephrologist before local or systemic treatment of uremic stomatitis.
- The oral lesions usually improve after hemodialysis.

Suggested Therapies

- High level of oral hygiene.
- Local mouthwashes with oxygen release agents such as hydrogen peroxide three to four times daily for 1–2 weeks.
- Chamomile mouthwash four to six times daily; keep in the mouth for about 5 minutes.
- Local antimycotics such as miconazole oral gel three to four times daily or nystatin oral suspension 5 mL three to four times daily if candidiasis is suspected.
- Artificial saliva substitutes for xerostomia.

References

Hovinga J, Roodvoets AP, Gaillard J. Some findings in patients with uremic stomatitis. *J Maxillofac Surg* 1975;3: 124–127.

Jaspers MT. Unusual oral lesions in a uremic patient. Review of the literature and report of a case. *Oral Surg Oral Med Oral Pathol* 1975;39:934–944.

Laskaris G. Color Atlas of Oral Diseases. 3rd edition, Thieme Verlag: Stuttgart, 2003.

McCreary CE, Flint SR, McCartan, et al. Uremic stomatitis mimicking oral hairy leukoplakia. *Oral Surg Oral Med Oral Pathol Oral Radiol Endod* 1997;83:350–355.

Verruca Vulgaris

■ Definition

Verruca vulgaris or the common wart is a benign skin lesion that rarely involves the oral mucosa.

■ Etiology

HPV types 1, 2, and 4, and rarely other strains are frequently the cause.

■ Main Clinical Features

Oral lesions occur most frequently as a result of autoinoculation from lesions on the hands or fingers. The lesions are more common in children.

Oral Lesions

- Small, sessile, well-defined exophytic growth with a cauliflower appearance and white or normal color
- Lesions are painless and can be single or multiple
- Lips, buccal mucosa, tongue, and gingiva are more frequently involved

Skin Lesions

- Exophytic, dome-shaped papules or nodules
- The lesions are usually painless
- They are most frequently located on the fingers, dorsum of hands, knees, and elbows. Nail involvement is also common

■ Diagnosis

The clinical diagnosis may be confirmed by histopathologic examination. In-situ hybridization may also be useful in difficult cases.

■ Differential Diagnosis

- Papilloma
- Condyloma acuminatum
- Verruciform xanthoma
- Focal epithelial hyperplasia
- Sialadenoma papilliferum
- Early verrucous carcinoma

■ Treatment

Basic Guidelines

- There is no specific antiviral therapy.
- The treatment of oral lesions should be followed by the treatment of skin lesions.
- Cutaneous lesions are sometimes self-limiting.
- Treatment of cutaneous common warts must be provided by a dermatologist.

Suggested Therapies

- Conservative surgical excision of oral lesions is the treatment of choice.
- Electrosurgery or CO_2 laser or cryotherapy may also be used.
- 5 % Imiquimod cream is used only for lesions on the vermilion border and the skin of the lips. Apply once daily on three alternate days per week for about 8–10 weeks.

Future Therapies

Specific antiviral agents and vaccination.

References

Benton EC. Therapy of cutaneous warts. *Clin Dermatol* 1997;15:449–453.

Beutner KR, Spruance SL, Hougham AJ, et al. Treatment of genital warts with an immunoresponse modifier (imiquimod). *J Am Acad Dermatol* 1998;38:230–239.

Laskaris G. *Color Atlas of Oral Diseases*, 3rd edition. Thieme Verlag: Stuttgart, 2003.

Muzio G, Massone C, Rebora A. Treatment of non-genital warts with topical imiquimod 5 % cream. *Eur J Dermatol* 2002;12:347–349.

Verrucous Carcinoma

■ Definition

Verrucous carcinoma is a relatively rare low-grade variant of oral squamous cell carcinoma.

■ Etiology

The etiology is unknown. Tobacco usage and HPV (types 16, 18, and 33) seem to play an important role in the development of the neoplasm.

■ Main Clinical Features

- Slowly growing, white exophytic mass with papillomatous or warty surface
- The lesion is usually painless and well demarcated
- Size ranges from 1 cm to several centimeters if left untreated
- The buccal mucosa, gingiva, and palate are the most common sites of involvement
- Neoplasms more frequently affect individuals older than 60 years

■ Diagnosis

The diagnosis should be confirmed by a biopsy and histopathologic examination.

■ Differential Diagnosis

- Squamous cell carcinoma
- Verrucous leukoplakia
- Verrucous hyperplasia
- Hairy leukoplakia
- Papilloma
- Verruciform xanthoma
- White sponge nevus
- Cinnamon contact stomatitis

■ Treatment

Basic Guidelines

- Early diagnosis and treatment usually cures the disease.
- Cessation of smoking.

Suggested Therapies

- Surgical excision is the treatment of choice with usually excellent results.
- Radiotherapy combined with chemotherapy is the next most preferred treatment when surgery is not indicated in advanced disease.
- Radiotherapy alone should be avoided as highly malignant transformation can occasionally occur.
- Chemotherapy alone or in combination with surgery may also be used as an alternative treatment in patients with extensive oral verrucous carcinoma.

References

Impola U, Uitto V, Hietanen J, et al. Differential expression of matrilysin-1 (MMP-7), 92 kD gelatinase (MMP-9), and metalloelastase (MMP-12) in oral verrucous and squamous cell cancer. *J Pathol* 2004;202:14–22.

Koch BB, Trask DK, Hoffman HT, et al. National survey of head and neck verrucous carcinoma: patterns of presentation, care, and outcome. *Cancer* 2001;92:110–120.

Salesiotis A, Soong R, Diasio RB, et al. Capecitabine induces rapid, sustained response in two patients with extensive oral verrucous carcinoma. *Clin Cancer Res* 2003;9:580–585.

Syrjanen S. Human papillomavirus infections and oral tumors. *Med Microbiol Immunol (Berl)* 2003;192:123–128.

Yeh CJ. Treatment of verrucous hyperplasia and verrucous carcinoma by shave excision and simple cryosurgery. *Int J Oral Maxillofac Surg* 2003;32:280–283.

Yoshimura Y, Mishima K, Obara S, et al. Treatment modalities for oral verrucous carcinomas and their outcomes: Contribution of radiotherapy and chemotherapy. *Int J Clin Oncol* 2001;6:192–200.

Wegener Granulomatosis

Definition

Wegener granulomatosis is a rare chronic granulomatous disease characterized by necrotizing granulomatous lesions of both upper and lower respiratory tracts, glomerulonephritis, and generalized focal necrotizing vasculitis.

Etiology

The etiology is unknown, although an immunologic mechanism is probably involved in the pathogenesis.

Main Clinical Features

The disease usually presents with respiratory signs and symptoms following by renal and other organ involvement. The oral lesions are fairly common and occasionally may be the initial and only sign for a long time. Fever, malaise, and weight loss are early and common symptoms.

Oral Lesions

Solitary or multiple painful ulcers surrounded by an inflammatory zone. Vegetating gingival enlargement is an early sign

Skin Lesions

Skin involvement occurs in half of the patients and is characterized by papules, petechiae, plaques, and ulcers

Respiratory Tract Lesions

Cough, dyspnea, hemoptysis. Nasal congestion, sinusitis, otitis media, mastoiditis

Renal Lesions

Glomerulonephritis

Other Organ Involvement

Ocular, cardiac, joint, and neurologic manifestations may occur

Diagnosis

The clinical diagnosis should be confirmed by biopsy and histopathologic examination, and the positive serum test for antineutrophil cytoplasmic antibodies (ANCA). Chest radiographs and CT, blood count and urinalysis may also be helpful.

Differential Diagnosis

- Malignant granuloma
- Non-Hodgkin lymphoma
- Leukemias
- Cryoglobulinemia
- Giant cell arteritis
- Polyarteritis nodosa
- Other vasculitides
- Systemic lupus erythematosus
- Tuberculosis
- Systemic mycoses

Treatment

Basic Guidelines

- The two principal aims of the treatment of Wegener granulomatosis are: first to limit the extent and severity of permanent organ damage by controlling the disease promptly, and secondly, to minimize the short- and long-term morbidity that is often the result of treatment.
- Rheumatologists and internists must undertake treatment of the disease.
- Disease localized and limited to the oral mucosa may be treated by a specialist stomatologist in collaboration with the rheumatologist.

Suggested Therapies

Systemic Treatment

Corticosteroids and Immunosuppressive Drugs

Prednisolone 0.5–1 mg/kg per day and cyclophosphamide 1.5–2 mg/kg per day are the mainstay of initial treatment and usually control the disease in about 1–1.5 months time. Azathioprine 1–2 mg/kg per day may also be used in association with prednisolone and cyclophosphamide as initial treatment. The combination of methotrexate, 20 mg/week, and prednisolone or prednisone is effective, particularly for patients who do not have immediately life-threatening disease.

Trimethoprim-sulfamethoxazole

This has been used in the treatment of limited Wegener granulomatosis with success. It is also effective for maintaining remission.

Topical Treatment

Painful oral lesions may be helped by topical steroids (0.1 % triamcinolone acetonide or 0.05 % clobetasol) in an adhesive base (Orabase) or with intralesional injection of corticosteroids retard. Topical anesthetics such as 5 % lidocaine (Xylocaine) ointment or viscous lidocaine may also reduce the pain for short time. The topical treatment of oral lesions is carried out in conjunction with the systemic treatment.

Alternative and Future Therapies

These include antilymphocytic monoclonal antibodies and anti-TNF-alpha antibodies. Plasmapheresis can be considered when pharmacological options are exhausted.

References

Koldingsnes W, Nossent JC. Baseline features and initial treatment as predictors of remission and relapse in Wegener's granulomatosis. *J Rheumatol* 2003;30:80–88.

Sangle S, Karim MY, Hughes GR, D'Cruz DP. Sulphamethoxazole-trimethoprim in the treatment of limited paranasal Wegener's granulomatosis. *Rheumatology (Oxford)* 2002;41:589–590.

Thomas-Golbanov C, Sridharan S. Novel therapies in vasculitis. *Expert Opin Invest Drugs* 2001;10:1279–1289.

Regan MJ, Hellmann DB, Stone JH. Treatment of Wegener's granulomatosis. *Rheum Dis Clin North Am* 2001;27:863–886.

Sambrook P. Isolated maxillary Wegener's granulomatosis: a case report and literature review. *Ann R Austral Coll Dent Surg* 2000;15:164–165.

Part II
Drugs

N. Choulis

■ Introduction

Drugs are life-saving entities used to gain increased control over the quality of our lives—to live better and longer. Drugs, for example antibiotics, save the lives of thousands. Thus the dentist and oral specialist who are concerned with the health and diagnosis of diseases of the mouth and the head and neck are able to treat many diseases, utilizing the arsenal of drugs available.

The establishment of a drug's specificity and therapeutic efficacy is a difficult task which requires prolonged pharmacological, toxicological, and clinical studies for the product to be a safe and effective treatment option for the disease it was intended to cure. The therapeutic index of drugs is of particular significance for the drugs employed in dentistry since safety per se is of paramount importance in dental practice. This aspect assumes even greater significance in the light of the clinical training and experience of the dentist in the management of acute allergic or toxic drug reactions, which is considerably less than that of the physician.

Finally, the distribution, fate, and elimination of drugs are of much relevance to dentistry, along with the advantages and hazards of drugs excreted into the saliva. For example, the presence of broad-spectrum antibiotics in the saliva exerts considerable influence on the oral microbial flora. An alteration of the oral microbial flora can affect caries incidence or trigger the onset of oral diseases such as candidiasis.

This part of the book deals with some of the categories of drug such as antimicrobials, antifungals, antiviral agents, corticosteroids, immunosuppressives, nonsteroidal anti-inflammatory agents, and antihistamines. The preparation, dosage, pharmacokinetics, side effects, possible interactions, and clinical uses of each category of drug are discussed.

■ Antimicrobial Agents

Antimicrobial agents are drugs used for treating infections caused by bacteria. Antibiotics have traditionally been divided into bacteriostatic, which reversibly inhibit the growth of susceptible microorganisms, and bactericidal, which kill the organisms. However, an antibiotic which is bactericidal in some concentrations may behave as a bacteriostatic agent in lower concentrations.

The sensitivity of a given strain of microorganism to an antibiotic is measured by the minimum inhibitory concentration (MIC), that is, the lowest concentration of antibiotic which will inhibit the growth of that strain of microorganism under controlled conditions. Similarly, the term minimum bactericidal concentration (MBC) can also be used. This is the lowest concentration of antibiotic that totally suppresses the growth of organisms when subcultured onto antibiotic-free media.

Sensitivity and resistance to antibiotic action are two important parameters to be considered. Sensitivity is tested by two methods, the dilution method, which determines the action of an antibiotic on a given bacterial strain, and the disk diffusion method, which simultaneously tests the inhibitory effect of various antibiotics.

Antibiotics should not be used indiscriminately and their choice should be based on a number of factors. Before choosing an antibiotic it is advisable to consider whether such treatment is essential. Ideally, the choice of antibiotic is based on the results of sensitivity tests interpreted with reference to the response achieved with the indicated treatment in similar conditions. When it is necessary to treat patients before sensitivity tests have been carried out, the drug therapy should be broad enough to cover all the pathogens that are suspected of causing the infection.

Antibiotics are divided into two broad categories: those that can be prescribed by all physicians, such as penicillins, ampicillin, amoxicillin, cefotaxime, metronidazole, gentamicin etc; and those that require the approval of a physician specializing in infectious diseases. This category of antibiotics includes second- and third-generation cephalosporins, newer quinolones, and some aminoglycosides etc. Moreover, the use of antibiotics should be restricted to those that are safe with minimal local or systemic side effects.

Penicillins

Penicillin, the first antibiotic to be used therapeutically, was originally developed as a mixture of penicillins known as F, G, X, and K, from the mold *Penicillium notatum.* Better yields were achieved from *P. chrysogenum* and benzylpenicillin (penicillin G) was selectively produced by adding the precursor, phenylacetic acid, to the fermentation medium. "Penicillin" is now used as a generic term for the entire group of natural and semisynthetic penicillins, which are still widely used; they are generally well tolerated, apart from hypersensitivity reactions, and are usually bactericidal by virtue of their inhibitory action on bacterial cell wall synthesis.

Pharmacokinetics

Penicillin G, as its alkaline (sodium or potassium) salt, is absorbed rapidly, particularly by the i. m. route. The drug can also be administered intravenously when a high concentration in blood is required. Absorption of the injected penicillin can be slowed by using "depot" preparations—a single dose of 300 000 U of procaine penicillin injected in an aqueous suspension form maintains therapeutic blood levels from 12 hours to 24 hours, or even 24–48 hours when oil is used as the excipient. On the other hand, absorption of penicillin G from the gastrointestinal tract is incomplete and irregular. To obtain sustainable results, equivalent to the parenteral, doses of three to five times are required. Penicillins are excreted mainly into the urine, mostly by tubular secretion. The normal plasma half-life of penicillin G is about three-quarters of an hour.

Side Effects and Interactions

Penicillins are considered to be nontoxic compounds, although many patients develop hypersensitivity reactions. The frequency of reactions to penicillins, particularly serious allergic reactions, has often led oral physicians to use antibiotics other than penicillins. Nevertheless, all available penicillins find some use in dental practice, with the exception of penicillin G-benzanthine.

Side Effects of Penicillins

General: Skin rash, nephropathy, angioedema, rare pericarditis, hepatotoxicity, anaphylactic reactions
Oral penicillins: Nausea, vomiting, diarrhea
High doses of penicillins: Neurotoxicity, nerve damage

The most commonly used penicillins, their preparation and doses/dosages are summarized in Table 2.**1**.

Cephalosporins

The cephalosporins are semisynthetic antibiotics derived from cephalosporin C, a natural antibiotic produced by the mold *Cephalosporium acremonium.* The active nucleus, 7-aminocephalosporanic acid, is very closely related to the penicillin nucleus. Cephalosporins of all generations are of beneficial use in dentistry.

Cephalosporins are bactericidal and, similar to penicillins, they act by inhibiting synthesis of the bacterial cell wall. The most widely used system of classification of cephalosporins is the "generations." Cephalothin was the first cephalosporin to have become available and is representative of the first-generation cephalosporins.

The third-generation cephalosporins, sometimes referred to as extended-spectrum cephalosporins are even more stable against hydrolysis by β-lactamases than cefamandole and cefuroxime. Compared with the earlier generations of cephalosporins they have greater potency and a wider spectrum of activity against Gram-negative organisms including most clinically important Enterobacteriaceae. They are generally less active against Gram-positive or-

Table 2.**1** Preparations and dosages of penicillins

Drug	Preparation	Dosage/dose
Amoxicillin	Capsules: 250 and 500 mg Oral suspensions: 500 mg/mL, 125 and 250 mg/5 mL Chewable: 125 and 250 mg	Oral: Adults and children over 20 kg: 250–500 mg/8 h up to 4.5 g/day Infants: 50 mg/8 h Children, 6–8 kg: 50–100 mg/8 h Children, 8–20 kg: 7–13 mg/kg every 8 h
Amoxicillin in combination with clavulanate		Amoxicillin: 500 mg Clavulanate potassium: 25 mg
Ampicillin	Capsules: 250 and 500 mg Oral suspensions: 100 mg/mL, 125, 250, 500 mg/5 mL	Oral: Adults and children over 20 kg: 250–500 mg/ 6 h Infants and children under 20 kg: 12.5–25 mg/kg every 6 h to 16.7–33 mg/kg every 8 h

ganisms compared with the first-generation agents.

The peroral bioavailability of cephalosporins fluctuates from 15% to 86% with a half-life of 0.5–6.5 hours. They are eliminated by glomerular and tubular secretion.

Side Effects of Cephalosporins

- Hypersensitivity in the form of fever, urticaria, angioneurotic edema, anaphylaxis, thrombocytopenia, nephritis
- Contraindicated if history of previous reaction to penicillins
- Pain and abscess at the site of intramuscular injection, nausea, vomiting, diarrhea, loose stools, abdominal pain, heartburn

Some commonly used representatives of cephalosporins and their doses are given in Table 2.**2**.

Tetracyclines

The tetracyclines are a group of antibiotics, originally derived from certain *Streptomyces* species having the same tetracyclic nucleus, naphthacene, and similar properties. Unlike the penicillins and aminoglycosides they are usually bacteriostatic at concentrations achieved in the body and act similarly to the aminoglycosides, i.e., by interfering with protein synthesis in susceptible organisms.

Tetracyclines all have a broad spectrum of activity which includes Gram-positive and Gram-negative bacteria, chlamydiae, rickettsiae, mycoplasmas, and spirochetes, but the emergence of resistant strains and the development of other antimicrobial agents have reduced their value. The extent of gastrointestinal absorption of these drugs is 58–100%. Tetracyclines complex with bivalent and trivalent metal ions, so that their absorption is greatly impaired by calcium, magnesium, and aluminum-containing antacids and by iron preparations. If possible, such drugs should be withheld during tetracycline therapy or at least not administered within 1 hour before or after the tetracycline. Food, especially milk products or other high-calcium foods, also interferes with oral absorption of tetracyclines. Phosphate appears to improve absorption, in part by removing calcium. All tetracyclines are bound to plasma proteins. Renal excretion is the principal mode of elimination, though minocycline is excreted mostly in the bile and more than 50% of doxycycline is metabolized and/or excreted into the colon. Preparations and dosages of tetracyclines are given in Table 2.**3**.

Side Effects of Tetracyclines

- Gastrointestinal disturbances, deposition in bones and teeth, anti-anabolic effects, fatty changes in the liver, photosensitivity
- Intramuscular injections are painful

Table 2.**2** Preparations and doses of cephalosporins

Drug	Preparation	Dose
Cefazolin sodium	Injectable: 500 mg/50 mL, 1g/50 mL Powder (in sterile form): 250 mg, 500 mg, 1 g, 10 g	Adults: i. v., i. m., 1 g/6–8 h Infants over 1 month: 6.25–25 mg/kg every 6–8 h
Cefoxitin sodium	Powder for injection in 1,2,10 g and solutions 1 and 2 g/50 mL	Adults: 1–2 g/4–8 h Infants over 3 months and children: 13.3–24.7 mg/kg every 4 h or 20–40 m/kg every 6 h
Cefotaxime sodium	Powder for injection in 0, 5, 1, 2 g	1–2 g/4 h i. v. or i. m. Children: 8.3–30 mg/kg every 4 h

Table 2.**3** Preparations and dosage of tetracyclines

Drug	Preparation	Dose
Tetracycline and tetracycline HCl	Suspension: 125 mg/5 mL Capsules: 100, 250, 500 mg Injections: 100, 250 mg i. v. injections: 250, 500 mg Tablets: 250, 500 mg	Injections (not in children under 8 years): 250–500 mg/6 h, 500 mg–1g/12 h HCl form same as tetracycline Adults and children over 8 years: i. m.: 100 mg/8 h, 150 mg/12 h, 250 mg/once a day i. v.: 250–500 mg/once
Oxytetracycline and oxytetracycline HCl	Injections: 50, 125 mg/mL Capsules: 125, 500 mg Tablets: 250 mg Injections: 250 and 500 mg	Injectable: 100 mg/8 h, 150 mg/12 h or 250 mg/once For children over 8 years: 5–8.3 mg/kg every 8 h or 7.5–12.5 mg/kg every 12 h HCl form: 250 mg/6 h orally For children over 8 years: 6.25 to 12.5 mg/kg every 6 h, i. v. 200–500 mg/12 h. Children (over 8) 5–10 mg/kg/12 h
Minocycline	Capsules, oral suspension, tablets, sterile (HCl form): 50 mg and 200 mg	Usual dose by either route: 200 mg/day in divided doses/12 h. Children: 4 mg/kg every 12 h followed by 2 mg/kg every 12 h.

- Should be avoided in pregnant women and in children
- Dizziness, vertigo, and pigmentation of the skin

Macrolides

The macrolides are a large group of antibiotics mainly derived from *Streptomyces* species. Their properties are very similar, and, in general, they have low toxicity. The macrolide antibiotics are bacteriostatic or bactericidal, depending on the concentration and the type of microorganism targeted and are thought to interfere with bacterial protein synthesis. Their antimicrobial spectrum is similar to that of benzylpenicillin but they are also active against such organisms as *Legionella pneumophila*, *Mycoplasma pneumoniae* and some rickettsiae and chlamydiae.

Erythromycin

Erythromycin is the only macrolide antibiotic to be widely used. It is absorbed variably after oral administration. In part this variability is the result of several types of enteric coating and in part due to biological variation. Absorption appears to be of zero reaction order, especially with higher doses. Food interferes with absorption and the antibiotic is destroyed by gastric acid. Peak plasma levels are attained in 1–4 hours, following which the concentration declines sharply by the fourth to the sixth hour. It is 73% bound to plasma proteins. The plasma half-life is 1.2–2 hours, though it may be up to 5–6 hours in cases of renal insufficiency.

Erythromycin is used as an alternative to penicillin, especially in patients who are allergic to the latter, and, similarly to tetracycline. Preparations and dosages are given in Table 2.**4**.

Side Effects of Erythromycin

- Gastrointestinal disturbances, skin reactions, reversible deafness (high doses), hepatotoxicity, irritation after topical administration
- Nausea, vomiting

Nitroimidazoles

The isolation of the antibiotic azomycin (2-nitroimidazole) from a streptomycete was achieved in 1953 and demonstration of its trichomonacidal properties led to the chemical synthesis and biological testing of many nitroimidazoles. One compound, 1-(b-hydroxyethyl)-2-methyl-5-nitroimidazole, now called metronidazole has especially high activity in vitro and in vivo against the anaerobic protozoa *Trichomonas vaginalis* and *Entamoeba histolytica*. Studies revealed that metronidazole had extremely useful clinical activity against a variety of anaerobic pathogens including both Gram-negative and Gram-positive bacteria, in addition to the protozoa. In dentistry the drug is used as an aid in periodontal therapy.

Metronidazole is available for oral, i.v., intravaginal, and topical use. Seventy-five percent of metronidazole is eliminated in urine following oral administration, the liver being the main site of metabolism.

Metronidazole is used for antiprotozoal therapy and particularly for the treatment of genital infections in both males and females. It is also used as an amebicide for all symptoms of amebiasis. It is also effective against a broad spectrum of anaerobic bacteria. The drug has excellent tissue penetration and reaches many organs. Side effects of metronidazole are outlined below and the preparations and doses are summarized in Table 2.**5**.

Side Effects of Metronidazole

- Headache, nausea, dry mouth, hairy tongue, metallic taste, vomiting, diarrhea

Table 2.**4** Preparation and dosage of erythromycin

Drug	Preparation	Dosage

Erythromycin	Enteric coated capsules: 125 and 250 mg
	Powders in 10, 25 and 100 mg, 2% solution
	Enteric coated tablets: 250 and 500 mg
		Oral:
		  Adults: 250 mg/6 h, 500 mg/6–12 h
		  Children: 7.5–25 mg/kg every 6 h or 15–50 mg/kg every 12 h

Table 2.**5** Preparations and doses of metronidazole

Drug	Preparation	Dosage

Metronidazole	Tablets: 200 and 500 mg
	I. V. infusion: 5 mg/mL
		Adults: 400–800 mg three times a day for 5–10 days
		Children:
		  1–3 years: 1/4 adult dose
		  3–7 years: 1/3 adult dose
		  7–10 years: 1/2 adult dose
		I. V.: 500 mg infused as 100 mL of a 5 mg/mL solution every 8 h

- When dizziness, convulsions, numbness of hands or legs, or urticaria is manifested the drug should be withdrawn

Antifungal Agents

The antifungal agents include a wide variety of chemical types of rather narrow antifungal spectra. Broad-spectrum antifungal agents are toxic and irritants, as expected from the prerequisite nonselectivity; however, the absorption of many of these agents through the epidermis is limited, and so they are employed in dermatological preparations. Not all antifungal agents are fungicidal; many are only fungistatic, and certain topical antifungal drugs owe their efficacy to a keratolytic action that causes sloughing of the stratum corneum with its entrained fungi.

The main group of azoles for systemic use are ketoconazole, fluconazole, itraconazole, and voriconazole. The main clinical uses of azoles are shown in Table 2.**6**.

Table 2.**6** Main clinical use of systemic azoles

Generic name	Diseases
Ketoconazole	Candidiasis, histoplasmosis, cryptococcosis, coccidioidomycosis, paracoccidioidomycosis
Fluconazole	Candidiasis, cryptococcosis, coccidioidomycosis
Itraconazole	Candidiasis, histoplasmosis, aspergillosis, blastomycosis, cryptococcosis, coccidioidomycosis, paracoccidioidomycosis
Voriconazole	Candidiasis, aspergillosis, histoplasmosis, coccidioidomycosis

Azole antifungal agents are the most popular in clinical use. Amphotericin B is a lipid formulation providing major reduction in renal toxicity.

The dosages and preparations of azoles are outlined in Table 2.**7**.

Side Effects of Azoles

Ketoconazole: Nausea, anorexia, vomiting, allergic rash, menstrual irregularities
Fluconazole: Nausea, vomiting, headache, skin rash, abdominal pain, diarrhea
Itraconazole: Gastrointestinal disturbances (doses of 400 mg), nausea, vomiting, hypertriglyceridemia, hypokalemia, rash, liver dysfunction. Doses over 400 mg are not recommended for long time use
Voriconazole: Rashes, transient abnormalities of liver enzymes, mild visual disturbances
Miconazole: Topical application causes burning, itching, irritation, headache, rash, diarrhea, anorexia, flashes, drowsiness

Echinocandins

Caspofugin

Caspofugin acetate is a water-soluble semisynthetic lipopeptide derivative of pneumocandin B, and is capable of inhibiting the formation of $\beta(1,3)$-D-glucans in the fungal cell wall. The drug has been found to be active, but only experimentally, in animals infected with *Candida albicans*. Currently, clinical trials are in progress in patients with systemic candidiasis.

Polyenes

Amphotericin B

Amphotericin is prepared by growing particular strains of *S. nodosus* in an appropriate medium followed by extraction and purification. It is poorly absorbed by the gastrointestinal tract and it is slowly excreted by the kidneys. The distribution half-life is 24–48 hours and the terminal half-life is about 15 days.

Amphotericin has the widest spectrum of antifungal activity compared with any other systemic drug. It is used intravenously for treating systemic fungal diseases. The main clinical uses and side effects of amphotericin B are given below, and the preparations and dosages are given in Table 2.**8**.

Table 2.7 Preparation and dosage/doses of azoles for oral diseases

Drug	Preparations	Dosage
Ketoconazole	2 % cream Oral suspensions: 100 mg/5 mL Tablets: 200 mg	Adult: 400 mg/day for 3–5 days Children over 2 years: 3.3–6.6 mg/kg per day
Fluconazole	Tablets: 50,100,200 mg Powder for suspension 10 and 40 mg/mL Injection solution (i. v.) 2 mg/mL	50–400 mg/day oral or i. v. Children: 3–6 mg/kg per day
Itraconazole	Capsules: 100 mg Injections, oral solution: 100 mg in 10 mL	100–200 mg/day for 6–15 days then 200 mg/day maintenance dose For seriously ill patients: 200 mg/twice a day (infusion) for 2 days followed by 200 mg/day for 12 days
Voriconazole	Film-coated tablets: 50 and 200 mg	Oral: Adult: 200–400 mg/12 h for 24 h, then 100–200 mg/12 h Not recommended for children under 2 years
Miconazole nitrate	Oral gel	125 mg four times daily
Clotrimazole	Troches: 100 mg	10 mg troches/5 times day for 2 weeks

Table 2.8 Preparation and dosage of amphotericin B

Drug	Preparation	Dosage
Amphotericin B	Injectable: 50 mg/15 mL	Adult dosing: 0.3–1.5 mg/kg IV qd. Give test dose of 1 mg IV over 20 minutes, increase by 5–10 mg/day.

Main Clinical Uses of Amphotericin B

- Systemic candidiasis
- Aspergillosis
- Cryptococcosis
- Histoplasmosis
- Blastomycosis
- Coccidioidomycosis
- Paracoccidioidomycosis

Side Effects of Amphotericin B

- Chills and fever, nausea and vomiting, diarrhea, abdominal "cramps", hemorrhagic gastroenteritis, dyspepsia, headache, vertigo, pain in the injected vein, thrombophlebitis, muscle and joint pains, anemia, purpura, hypertension, hypotension, cardiac arrest, ventricular fibrillation, skin rashes, hypokalemia, hypomagnesemia, renal damage, blood dyscrasias, loss of hearing, and other untoward effects

- It has been reported to cause pulmonary deterioration when given with blood products in granulocytopenia
- When given intrathecally it may cause grand mal convulsions, radiculitis, arachnoiditis, paralysis of the extremities, urinary retention, and other difficulties
- Because of the potential seriousness of its toxic effects, i. v. use should be primarily for hospitalized patients with progressive, potentially fatal infections; renal function should be monitored
- Hypokalemia may favor digitalis toxicity and sensitization to neuromuscular blocking drugs

■ Antiviral Agents

Drugs used in the therapy of or for protection against viral infections are known as antivirals. It is, however, necessary for the treatment to begin in the early stages of the infection for the drug to be effective. In general, they act by disrupting one of the many steps in viral infection and replication.

Viruses consist of either DNA or RNA enclosed in a protein coat. DNA viruses include poxviruses (smallpox), herpesviruses (chickenpox, herpes), adenoviruses (sore throat), hepadnaviruses (hepatitis B), and papillomavirus (warts). RNA viruses includes rubella virus (German measles), rhabdovirus (rabies), picornaviruses (polio, meningitis and colds), orthomyxoviruses (influenza), and paramyxoviruses (measles, mumps). The main clinical uses of systemic antivirals are presented in Table 2.**9**.

Side Effects of Antiviral Agents

Acyclovir:
● Intravenous: Local reactions, inflammation, pain, phlebitis, skin rashes
● Topical: Burning or erythema
● Oral: Rashes, gastrointestinal disturbances
Valacyclovir: Side effects and precautions similar to acyclovir
Famciclovir: Headache, nausea, diarrhea, urticaria, rash, hallucinations

Table 2.**9** Main clinical uses of systemic antivirals

Generic name	Diseases
Acyclovir	Primary herpetic gingivostomatitis, herpes zoster
Valacyclovir	Primary herpetic gingivostomatitis, herpes zoster
Famciclovir	Primary herpetic gingivostomatitis, herpes zoster

The preparations and doses of selective antiviral agents are given in Table 2.**10**.

Interferons

Interferons are potent cytokines that have antiviral, immunomodulating, and antiproliferative actions. They are produced in human or animal cells following exposure chiefly to viruses. They may also be manufactured through recombinant DNA technology.

Three major categories of human interferon are currently available: alpha, beta, and gamma. Interferon alpha, also known as leukocyte interferon, can be derived from those cells or through DNA technology. Interferon beta is also known as fibroblastic interferon after the cell type used for production, and interferon gamma is also known as immune interferon because it is derived from immunologically stimulated T-lymphocytes. The preparations and dosages are given in Table 2.**11**. Side effects of interferon mostly involve interferon alpha, particularly when given intramuscularly or intravenously.

Side Effects of Interferon

Interferon alpha and beta: Flu-like symptoms, fever, chills, myalgia, anorexia, alopecia, signs of altered liver function, renal failure, hypo- or hypertension, myocardial infarction, and stroke
Nasal administration: May cause mucosal irritation
Other side effects are:
● Dose-limiting toxicities of systemic administration are myelosuppression with granulocytopenia and thrombocytopenia

Table 2.**10** Preparation and dosage of antiviral agents

Drug	Preparations	Dosage
Acyclovir	Capsules: 200 mg	I. V:. 25 mg/mL can be further diluted to 5 mg/mL every 8 h for 5–7 days
	Powder reconstitute for i. v. use	Oral: 200 mg five times daily for 5 days. Can be increased to 400 mg/6 h
Valacyclovir	Capsules/tablets: 500 mg	Herpes simplex: 1000 mg twice a day for 10 days Herpes zoster (drug of choice): 1000 mg three times a day for 7 days
Famciclovir	Capsules/tablets: 250 mg	HIV-infected patients: 500 mg two times a day. Adult herpes zoster (recommended): 500 mg three times a day for 10 days

- Neurotoxicity, confusion, behavior disturbances
- Fatigue and weight loss
- Thyroiditis, cardiovascular effects, hypotension, tachycardia
- Elevation of hepatic enzymes and triglycerides. Also reduces the metabolism of various drugs

Table 2.**11** Preparation and dosages of interferon. Interferons are measured in units and characterized by their origin

Type of interferon	Units (U) in one ampoule
Human lymphoblastoid interferon alpha	25 000
Human leukocyte interferon alpha	12 000
Human recombinant interferon alpha-2a	9000
Human recombinant interferon alpha-2b	17 000
Human recombinant interferon alpha-1	8000
Human fibroblast interferon beta	15 000
Human recombinant interferon beta (Ser 17)	6000
Human interferon gamma	4000

■ Corticosteroids

Corticosteroids are effective against a large number of acute and chronic lesions of the oral mucosa. Topically applied corticosteroids have nearly no side effects. The main corticosteroids used systemically are hydroxy compounds, and the sodium salt of the phosphate or succinate ester provides water-soluble solutions for injection.

Corticosteroids are easily absorbed from the gastrointestinal tract and they also may be absorbed when administered topically and produce systemic effects. When in the blood circulation, only the unbound form has pharmacological effects. They are metabolized in the kidney and liver and excreted in the urine. Corticosteroids are used because of their anti-inflammatory and immunosuppressant glucocorticoid properties. During periods of stress, such as during or after surgery, the corticosteroid dosage must be increased. Although these drugs can be used in serious situations, generally it is advisable not to start corticosteroids until a conclusive diagnosis has been reached. The main clinical uses of systemic corticosteroids and their side effects are presented below.

Main Clinical Uses of Systemic Corticosteroids

- Pemphigus
- Sjögren syndrome
- Bullous pemphigoid
- Wegener granulomatosis
- Cicatricial pemphigoid
- Chronic ulcerative stomatitis
- Linear IgA disease
- Major aphthous ulcers
- Pemphigoid gestationis
- Eosinophilic ulcer
- Epidermolysis bullosa acquisita
- Pyostomatitis vegetans
- Erythema multiforme
- Lichen planus
- Toxic epidermal necrolysis
- Contact cheilitis
- Behçet disease
- Drug-induced oral ulcerations
- Sweet syndrome
- Dry socket
- Lupus erythematosus
- Melkersson–Rosenthal syndrome
- Scleroderma
- Orofacial granulomatosis

Side Effects of Long-Term Systemic Glucocorticosteroid Therapy

Gastrointestinal
- Esophagitis
- Peptic ulcer
- Pancreatitis
- Nausea
- Vomiting

Ophthalmic
- Cataract
- Glaucoma
- Hemorrhage
- Infection

Metabolic
- Hyperglycemia
- Hyperlipidemia
- Hypocalcemia

Cardiovascular
- Hypertension
- Edema
- Atherosclerosis

Musculoskeletal
- Osteoporosis
- Muscle atrophy
- Myopathy

Cutaneous
- Skin atrophy
- Acne
- Hirsutism
- Hyperpigmentation
- Hematoma
- Delay wound healing

Blood
- Leukocytosis
- Lymphopenia

Nervous system
- Mood changes
- Psychosis
- Peripheral neuropathy

Hormonal
- Amenorrhea
- Diabetes mellitus

Infections
- Virus
- Bacterial
- Mycoses

Table 2.**12** gives the preparations and dosages of corticosteroids

▮ Immunosuppressive Agents.

Immunosuppressive agents can attenuate the expression of at least one type of immune response. Immunosuppressive drugs comprise a number of classes of drug, such as antineoplastic, antimalarial, antibacterial, biological agents etc. Immunosuppressive agents are also used to prevent rejection of organ and bone marrow transplants. The main clinical uses and side effects of immunosuppressives are given below.

Main Clinical Uses of Immunosuppressive Agents

- Pemphigus
- Bullous pemphigoid
- Cicatricial pemphigoid
- Linear IgA disease
- Pemphigoid gestationis
- Wegener granulomatosis
- Lupus erythematosus

Side Effects of Immunosuppressive Agents

Azathioprine: Bone marrow suppression, thrombocytopenia, anemia, hepatotoxicity, gastrointestinal toxicity, pancreatitis

Cyclophosphamide: Bone marrow suppression, thrombocytopenia, anemia, hepatotoxicity, gastrointestinal toxicity, pancreatitis

Cyclosporine: Nephrotoxicity, hypertension, hyperkalemia, gastrointestinal disorders, acne, gingival overgrowth, tremor, hallucinations, anaphylactoid reactions

Mycophenolate mofetil: Gastrointestinal and hematologic disturbances, diarrhea, vomiting, leukopenia

Table 2.**12** Preparation and dosage of corticosteroids

Drug	Preparation	Dosage/dose
Cortisone acetate	Tablets Injectable	10–50 mg tablets 25 mg/mL in ampoules of 10 mL
Betamethasone	Tablets Injectable	0.5–5 mg/daily 4–20 mg
Dexamethasone	Tablets Injectable Inhalers Spray	0.5–5 mg daily 2–6 mg/kg 300 µg three times a day As required
Hydrocortisone	Tablets Injectable	I. V.: 10–40 mg/day (for rapid effect) Slowly 100–500 mg three to four times a day
Prednisolone	Tables (enteric coated): 2.5–5 mg Injectable: 25 mg/mL	Oral: 5–60 mg/day (divided doses) Parenteral: 4–60 mg/day Suspension: 25–100 mg/once a week

The preparations and dosages of this group of drugs are presented in Table 2.13. The latter is a macrolide antibiotic used for prophylaxis of solid-organ allograft rejection in a manner similar to cyclosporine and as rescue therapy in patients with rejection episodes.

Nonsteroidal Anti-inflammatory Agents

Drugs used to treat the symptoms of inflammation are known as anti-inflammatory agents, the most common being the nonsteroidal anti-inflammatory drugs (NSAIDs), which inhibit cyclooxygenase-1 (COX-1) and cyclooxygenase-2 (COX-2). The inhibition of COX-2 is partly responsible for the analgesic and anti-inflammatory actions, while inhibition of COX-1 leads to the side effects (i. e., gastric ulcer). The mechanism of action for the anti-inflammatory and analgesic effects of NSAIDs was only recently established.

Inflammation is caused by a number of factors, e. g., infectious agents, antigen–antibody interactions, or some sort of physical injury. On the basis of the differences in duration, type of cells, and mechanisms involved, inflammation can manifest as: a) the acute transient state, b) the delayed, subacute phase, and c) the chronic proliferative state.

The NSAIDs are mainly effective against pain of low-to-moderate intensity, e.g., dental pain. Chronic postoperative pain or pain arising from inflammation is also particularly well controlled by these drugs. However, these drugs only provide symptomatic relief from pain and inflammation associated with the disease, and they do not arrest the progression of pathological injury to tissue.

The most common side effects of these drugs are disturbances of the gastrointestinal system which can even result in bleeding; chronic use may cause nephropathy. Therefore, patients with peptic ulcers must avoid NSAIDs. In addition, NSAIDs may interact with anticoagulants, captopril, methotrexate, and triamterene. Some of the best known drugs with analgesic and anti-inflammatory properties are aspirin, diclofenac sodium, dipyrone, flufenamic acid, flurbiprofen, ibuprofen, indomethacin, ketoprofen, mefenamic acid, naproxen, niflumic acid, acetaminophen, phenazone, phenylbutazone, and piroxicam.

Antihistamines

Antihistamines are H_1-receptor antagonists stimulating gastric acid secretion. Drugs which antagonize H_2-receptors (H_2-receptor antagonists) inhibit gastric secretion.

Antihistamines are used for controlling allergic reactions that involve the oral tissues and structures. However, these drugs have not been used successfully in the management of postopera-

Table 2.**13** Preparation and dosage of immunosuppressive agents

Drug	Preparation	Dosage
Azathioprine	Injection Tablets: 50 mg	Single i. v. dose: 1–5 mg/kg per day Tablets: 50–100 mg/day
Cyclophosphamide	Injection Tablets: 25–50 mg	Single i. v. dose: 2–6 mg/kg per day also 10–15 mg/kg per week or 20–40 mg/kg per 15 days
Cyclosporine	Injection: 50 mg/mL Oral solution: 100 mg/mL Capsules: 25, 100 mg	I. V.: 1/3 of the oral dose Oral solution: taken with milk or orange juice twice at 14–18 mg/kg per day, for 4–12 h before transplantation continued for 1–2 weeks Maintenance dose 5–10 mg/kg per day Alternatively, capsules: 25 mg or 100 mg
Mycophenolate mofetil	Tablets: 250–500 mg	Oral: 1 g I. V.: twice daily (for renal transplant) Other uses under investigation currently, e. g., pemphigus vulgaris: 2–3 g/day

tive sequelae of oral surgery procedures (e.g., facial swelling, edema). Antihistamines are effective in relieving the symptoms of allergic rhinitis, conjunctivitis, systemic anaphylactic reactions, angioedema, and allergic skin disorders.

Antihistamines are given by mouth and should be taken with food or after eating to avoid gastric irritation. Injectable formulations are only given in cases of severe allergic reactions.

The most common side effects of antihistamines are sedation, nausea, vomiting, diarrhea, dry mouth, and hypotension. Overdose may be fatal, especially in infants and children.

▉ Other Drugs

The dentist's arsenal of drugs is not by far exhausted by the above mentioned categories of drug. Many other drugs, materials, and medical devices are used in the everyday practice of the professional dentist as they attempt to cure the vast array of lesions that arise in the mouth—ranging from traumatic ulcers to life-threatening malignancies. Many local disturbances and systemic diseases have oral manifestations, e.g., allergy, chemical burns, cysts, denture stomatitis, hyper- and hyposalivation, local infections, periodontitis, traumatic ulcers, tumors and neoplasms, hormonal aberrations, dermatologic diseases, hematologic disorders, osteoradionecrosis, maxillary sinusitis, stomatitis etc. Thus two other categories of agents deserve mention and are discussed briefly herein: anesthetics and hemostatics.

Anesthetics

Anesthetics are divided into local and topical anesthetics and general anesthetics. Local anesthetics are extensively used in dentistry and as the word indicates, applied locally to produce local anesthesia. At times, supplemental injections may be necessary: these are injections into bone, the dental pulp, periodontal ligament, and the palate. The most commonly used anesthetics are benzocaine, lidocaine, procaine, propoxycaine etc. Vasoconstrictors may also be required along with the local anesthetic solutions, and epinephrine, norepinephrine, and phenyle-

phrine are some of those recommended. Allergic reactions to the anesthetic drugs are not uncommon, especially of the fingers and face.

Hemostatic Agents

Blood is a frequent "byproduct," only second to pain, encountered during dental treatment (or the other way around for some people). There are many methods to stop the bleeding, e.g., pressure packing techniques, sutures, and cold applications. Epinephrine, aluminum and ferric chloride, collagen and thrombin are some of the recommended hemostatics. Epinephrine especially is effective in controlling capillary bleeding caused by filling materials inserted in the gum. However, care should be taken when the patient is undergoing anticoagulant therapy.

References

Argyropoulos SV, Nutt DJ. The use of benzodiazepines in anxiety and other disorders. *Eur Neuropsychopharmacol* 1999;9(suppl 6):S407–S412.

Christ M, Haseroth K, Falkenstein E, Wehling M. Nongenomic steroid actions: Fact or fantasy? *Vitam Horm* 1999;57:325–373.

Chrousos GP. The hypothalamic-pituitary-adrenal axis and immunomediated inflammation. *N Engl J Med* 1995; 332:1351–1362.

Clancio SG. *Remington's Pharmaceutical Sciences*, 18th edition, p. 1957. Mack Publishing Co: Easton PA, 1990.

DeJong RH. *Local Anesthetics.* Mosby: St Louis, MO, 1994.

Faulds D, Goa KL, Benfield P. Cyclosporin. A review of its pharmacodynamic and pharmacokinetic properties and therapeutic use in immunoregulatory disorders. *Drugs* 1993;45:953–1040.

Fife KH, Barbarash RA, Rudolf T, et al. Valaciclovir versus acyclovir in the treatment of first episode genital herpes infection. Results of an international, multicenter, double-blind, randomized clinical trial. The Valaciclovir International Herpes Simplex. Virus Study Group. *Sex Transm Dis* 1997;24:481–486.

Forsberg E, Pejler G, Ringvall M, et al. Abnormal mast cells in mice deficient in heparin-synthesized enzyme. *Nature* 1999;400:773–776.

Francois C, Duverlie G, Rebouillat D, et al. Expression of hepatitis C virus proteins interferes with the antiviral action of interferon independently of PRK-mediated control of protein synthesis. *J Virol* 2000;74:5587–5596.

Freeman CD, Klutman NE, Lamp KC. Metronidazole. A therapeutic review and update. *Drugs* 1997;54:679–708.

Ganapathy ME, Huang M, Wang H, et al. Valacyclovir: A substrate of the intestinal and renal peptide transporters PEPT1 and PEPT2. *Biochem Biophys Res Commun* 1998;246:470–475.

Gish RG. Standards of treatment in chronic hepatitis-C. *Semin Liver Dis* 1999;19(suppl 1):35–47.

Halloran PF. Immunosuppressive agents in clinical trials in transplantation. *Am J Med Sci* 1997;313:283–288.

Khanna A, Li B, Stenzel KH, Suthanthiran M. Regulation of new DNA synthesis in mammalian cells by cyclosporine. Demonstration of a transforming growth factor beta-dependent mechanism of inhibition of cell growth. *Transplantation* 1994;57:577–582.

Kimball JA, Peskovitz MD, Book BK, Normal DV. Reduced human IgG anti-ATGAM antibody formation in renal transplant recipients receiving mycophenolate mofetil. *Transplantation* 1995;60:1379–1383.

Kovac AL. Prevention and treatment of postoperative nausea and vomiting. *Drugs* 2000;59:213–243.

Lazarus HM, Belanger R, Candoni A, et al. Intravenous penciclovir for treatment of herpes simplex infections in immunocompromised patients: Results of a multicenter acyclovir-controlled trial. The Penciclovir Immunocompromised Study Group. *Antimicrob Agents Chemother* 1999;43:1192–1197.

Marichal P, Koymans L, Willemsens S, et al. Contribution of mutations in the cytochrome P450 14 alpha-dimethylase to azole resistance to *Candida albicans*. *Microbiology* 1999;145:2701–2713.

McKinsey DS, Wheat J, Cloud GA, et al. Itraconazole prophylaxis for fungal infections in patients with advanced human immunodeficiency virus infection: randomized, placebo-controlled, double-blind study. National Institute of Allergy and Infectious Diseases Mycoses Study Group. *Clin Infect Dis* 1999;28:1049–1056.

Noble S, Markham A. Cyclosporine. A review of the pharmacokinetic properties, clinical efficacy and tolerability of a microemulsion-based formulation (Neoral). *Drugs* 1995;50:924–941.

Nyquist AC, Gonzales R, Steiner JF, Sande MA. Antibiotic prescribing for children with colds, upper respiratory tract infections and bronchitis. *JAMA* 1998;279:875–877.

Pursley TJ, Blamquist IK, Abraham J, et al. Fluconasole-induced congenital abnormalities in three infants. *Clin Infect Dis* 1996;22:336–340.

Reeves RR, Carter OS, Rinkofsky HB, et al. Carisoprodol (SOMA): Abuse potential and physical unawareness. *J Addict Dis* 1999;18:51–56.

Rosenberg RD, Aird WC. Vascular-bed-specific hemostasis and hypercoagulable states. *N Engl J Med* 1999;340:1555–1564.

Rudolf U, Crestani F, Benke D, et al. Benzodiazepine actions mediated by specific gamma-aminobutyric acid (A) receptor subtypes. *Nature* 1999;401:796–800.

Sacks SL, Sasadeusz JJ, Shafran SD. Effects of long-term famciclovir treatment of sperm parameters in patients with recurrent genital herpes. 8th International Congress on Infectious Diseases, Boston, MA, Abstr. No 2202;1998.

Samuelson J. Why metronidazole is active against both bacteria and parasites. *Antimicrob Agents Chemother* 1999;43:1533–1541.

Seibert K, Zhang Y, Leahy K, et al. Distribution of Cox-1 and Cox-2 in normal and inflamed tissues. *Adv Exp Med Biol* 1997;400A:167–170.

Simon LS, Weaver AL, Graham DY, et al. Antiinflammatory and upper gastrointestinal effects of celecoxib in rheumatoid arthritis; a randomized controlled trial. *JAMA* 1999;282:1921–1928.

Simons FE, Simons KJ. The pharmacology and use of H_1-receptor antagonist drugs. *N Engl J Med* 1994;330:1663–1670.

Smith AJ, Nissan A, Lanonette NM, et al. Prokinetic effect of erythromycin after colorectal surgery: Randomized, placebo-controlled, double-blind study. *Dis Colon Rectum* 2000;43:333–337.

Wagstaff AJ, Bryson HM, Forscarnet A. A reappraisal of its antiviral activity, pharmacokinetic properties and therapeutic use in immunocompromised patients with viral infections. *Drugs* 1994;48:199–226.

Walsh TJ, Hiemenz JW, Seibel NL, et al. Amphotericin-B lipid complex for invasive fungal infections. Analysis of safety and efficacy of 556 cases. *Clin Infect Dis* 1998;26:1383–1396.

White MH, Bowden RA, Sandler ES, et al. Randomised double-blind clinical trial of amphotericin-B colloidal dispersion vs amphotericin B in the empirical treatment of fever and neutropenia. *Clin Infect Dis* 1998;27:296–302.

Wong-Beringer A, Jacobs RA, Gugliemo BJ. Lipid formulations of amphotericin-B clinical efficacy and toxicities. *Clin Infect Dis* 1998;27:603–618.

Yoshida H, Shiratori Y, Moriyama M, et al. Interferon therapy reduces the risk of hepatocellular carcinoma: national surveillance program of cirrhotic and noncirrhotic patients with chronic hepatitis C in Japan. IHIT Study Group. Inhibition of Hepatocarcinogenesis by Interferon Therapy. *Ann Intern Med* 1999;131:174–181.

Part III
Laser Therapy

G. E. Romanos

Laser Applications for the Treatment of Oral Mucosal Lesions

▩ Introduction

Modern surgical treatment of oral diseases is enhanced by the benefits of minimally invasive surgical techniques, such as laser therapy. The laser light is able to cut, coagulate, or ablate tissues by its high-power density.

LASER is an acronym for "light amplification by stimulated emission of radiation," that is, high-power light concentrated in a focused area—the target tissue. The laser light has several characteristic features:

- It is *coherent*, which means that the light is directed over a long distance without divergence, in contrast to sun or flash light.
- It is *collimated*, which means that the laser light can be concentrated in the target tissue with the light with the highest energy directed at the focus (spot).
- It is *monochromatic*, which means that it has only one wavelength.

The main part of the laser unit is the active medium. It is the "brain" of the whole system where electrons are activated for the emission of photons. Depending on the active medium, lasers can be classified into following categories:

- lasers using solid active media (crystals), i.e., Er:YAG, Nd:YAG, Ho:YAG lasers
- lasers using fluids, i.e., the dye lasers
- lasers using gases, i.e., CO_2, He:Ne, argon
- lasers using semiconductors (diodes), i.e., diode lasers.

Lasers can further be distinguished on the basis of their power setting, "soft" lasers use a power setting of mW to W (Watts) and "hard" (surgical) lasers between W and kW. In addition, all laser units are classified according to the safety level of the laser (safety classes 1, 2, 3A, 3B, and 4) and according to the damage caused to vital tissues (skin, retina), i.e., reversible or irreversible. Most lasers used in medical applications belong to class 3B or 4 and, for the same reason, in practices where lasers are used, a laser safety officer (certified in laser safety) is responsible for laser safety measures.

▩ Laser–Tissue Interactions

The specific interaction between the laser and the tissues depends on several physical parameters (power, power density, energy, pulses, frequency, exposure time, focal spot size etc.), tissue consistency and, last but not least, the wavelength of the laser. Most important among the optical properties of the tissues are the reflection, absorption, scattering, and transmission of light during laser irradiation. Currently, laser–tissue interactions are classified in five categories: photochemical interactions, photothermal effects, photoablation, plasma-induced ablation, and photodisruption.

Photochemical interactions occur when using lasers with low-power densities and long exposure times. The laser light induces chemical effects and production of molecules in the tissues. Such phenomena are of great importance in the field of photodynamic therapy (PDT), where a photosensitizer is injected into the body and activated after laser irradiation. This technique has beneficial effects in the treatment of cancer. Another phenomenon based on photochemical interaction is biostimulation. This term was used loosely and only recently has been explained on the basis of several experimental studies. Laser has a biostimulating effect on tissues, that is, after laser irradiation the healing mechanisms are accelerated and vascularization and collagen synthesis may be enhanced and postoperative pain reduced. Thus, for evidence for such effects reproducible experiments and standardized treatment protocols are necessary rather than anecdotal explanations.

Several *photothermal* laser–tissue interactions can be distinguished depending on the power density used. Specifically, coagulation, vaporization, carbonization, and melting are thermal phenomena with clinical advantages for the clinician. The tissue has to be effectively coagulated during surgery. With the use of special laser systems it is possible today to seal the blood vessels at the wound margins without causing extensive damage to the surrounding tissues. The coagulation properties are dependent on the laser parameters, especially the wavelength used. Vaporization is another photothermal phenomenon where water vapor builds up in the air under pressure. When the temperature increases or the power (or energy) applied is too high, carbon deposits on the tissue surface change the color of the tissue. There is more tissue necrosis, and therefore, the wound healing processes are slower.

Melting is a dramatic effect of the laser light as the high-energy light density is able to "breakdown" the tissue. The surface of a tooth or an implant can be extensively melted in a short time using different wavelengths and laser parameters. This phenomenon is different from *photoablation*, in which sufficient power is supplied to the ultraviolet photons to break the binding chains between the molecules in an extremely short time. This makes possible precise ablation of the tissue in pulses with very short durations (10–100 nsec) without any evidence of thermal damage, such as coagulation or vaporization. With even smaller pulse durations (picoseconds [psec] to femtoseconds [fsec]), different effects of clinical interest and diagnostic importance will be possible in the future.

Plasma-induced ablation involves removal of tissue without thermal or mechanical damage using appropriate laser parameters. The idea is to ablate the tissues by ionizing plasma formation using pulse durations in the psec to fsec range. Application of plasma-induced ablation in corneal surgery and dental caries therapy may be possible in the future.

Finally, *photodisruption* is a combination of plasma formation, shock wave generation, cavitation, and jet formation using higher pulse energies and pulse durations in the range of nsec to fsec. Photodisruption may be used to mechanically split tissues as in lithotripsy and lens capsulotomy.

Laser light emission is higher and completely different in blood vessels compared with connective tissue matrix with the wavelengths used with Nd:YAG (1064 nm), argon (488 nm or 514 nm), or diode (980 nm or 810 nm) lasers. The laser–tissue interactions are different when the laser wavelength is 10 600 nm (CO_2) or 2940 nm (Er:YAG laser).

Similarly, the CO_2 or the Er:YAG laser is better absorbed by the superficial soft tissues, especially by light-colored lesions, while absorption by pigmented lesions is reduced. In addition, Er:YAG laser light emission is higher in enamel, dentin, bone, or other calcified tissues but does not have high penetration depth in comparison with other laser systems (CO_2, Nd:YAG, diode, Argon, dye, Ho:YAG etc.). The depth of penetration of the Nd:YAG laser is 3–4 mm compared with the CO_2 laser, which only penetrates and affects superficial layers to a depth of 0.1–0.3 mm.

■ Laser Applications in Oral Medicine

The differences in the properties of the different laser wavelengths are the main reasons for the variety of clinical effects of lasers seen in dentistry. In this section the clinical indications of the different laser systems in the treatment of oral mucosal lesions are presented. The advantages, disadvantages, and complications of the different established dental laser units will be discussed to give some guidelines to the clinician. On the basis of published evidence as well as my own clinical experience, an analysis of the treatment of the most important oral lesions encountered in daily practice will be presented.

When treating oral soft-tissue lesions two different techniques can be used: excision or ablation. For the first choice the laser beam is focused in a way that excises the tissue. In ablative techniques the tissue is removed and vaporized layer by layer without the possibility of histological examination of a biopsy. In any event, in case of tissue removal with a laser system, a special informed consent has to be given to the oral pathologist to explain better the possible structural changes. Because the surface of most oral tissues has a high water content, the CO_2 laser is indicated in most cases of soft-tissue surgery. This allows a relatively precise line of incision in association with appropriate coagulation properties. Table **1** gives the indications of the different laser wavelengths in oral medicine.

Benign Tumors

For the removal of soft-tissue tumors (fibromas, adenomas, lipomas etc.) the CO_2 laser can be

Table **3.1** The various laser wavelengths and their indications in oral medicine

Laser	Lesion
CO_2, diode, Nd:YAG, Er:YAG	Benign tumors
CO_2, diode, Nd:YAG	Mucocoeles
Nd:YAG, argon, diode	Hemangiomas
CO_2	Drug-induced gingival overgrowth
CO_2, Er:YAG, Nd:YAG, diode, dye, Argon	Tattoos and pigmented lesions
CO_2, Er:YAG	Leukoplakia
CO_2, diode, Er:YAG	Peri-implant gingival overgrowth

easily used with a noncontact, focused beam in continuous wave mode. In most cases, depending on the laser unit being used, a power setting between 2 W and 6 W is sufficient for most minor surgical procedures. For large tumors of the oral cavity, CO_2 lasers in an ultrapulse mode can be more advantageous for the specialist oral maxillofacial surgeon. In all cases a noncontact beam is used and the delivery system that transfers the laser energy to the target tissue is either an articulated arm or a hollow guide. These delivery systems have some advantages and disadvantages. The hollow guide is very flexible, does not have any mirrors in its volume allowing reflection, and therefore light transfers without any loss of energy. In contrast, articulated arms allow reflection in the system (with no loss of energy) but less flexibility in their application.

For removal of small soft-tissue tumors in the oral cavity the application of fiber-delivery laser systems, such as the diode (810 nm and 980 nm) or the Nd:YAG laser can also be used. Because of the higher penetration depth of the wavelengths of these lasers, the direction of the laser light during surgery has to be under precise control in order to avoid necrosis or other complications of the surrounding healthy tissues. Such complications can be observed when the lasers are incorrectly applied near healthy periodontal tissues. The laser beam will be in contact with the tissue to excise the tumor and to make possible the histological examination. The use of noncontact devices results in only coagulation of the tumor.

This produces changes in the tissue structure after coagulation of the blood vessels and sometimes presents problems for the pathologist. The coagulation properties of these devices are excellent and therefore they can be used in the treatment of patients with systemic bleeding disorders.

Mucoceles

Small cystic lesions of the minor salivary glands can be excised using different laser wavelengths. The CO_2 laser is the chief representative for such surgical procedures, but lasers with glass fiberoptics allow the practitioner to carry out an easy and painless surgical excision. The coagulation properties of the diode and Nd:YAG lasers are sufficient to achieve hemostasis and for that reason sutures are not necessary after surgery. In most cases the use of low-power settings between 3 W and 5 W is not associated with any complication, such as scar tissue formation or recurrence.

Hemangiomas

It is of special interest to the clinician to be able to remove subcutaneous hemangiomas of the face as well as of the oral cavity and the perioral regions without complications (i.e., bleeding). Two possibilities have to be considered. The classic method of excision is with a scalpel or CO_2, diode, Er:YAG, or Nd:YAG laser to be able to study the histology of the tumor. The second possibility is coagulation and vaporization of the hemangioma. In this technique, a laser system with excellent coagulation properties is of great importance. We use the Nd:YAG, the diode (980 nm) or the argon laser in order to coagulate sufficiently. In our method of treatment, we place an ice cube on the surface of the hemangioma and irradiate the tumor without touching the tumor surface. The glass fiber has to penetrate the ice cube and after irradiation it is possible to carry out continuous coagulation of the lesion. The coagulation results in a visible change in the color. For big hemangiomas repeat laser irradiation 2–3 weeks later is necessary. The tumor size is reduced significantly and after vaporization there are no aesthetic or functional complications. We have used this surgical method for coagulation of hemangiomas and telangiectasias for many years, and we recommend the application of the Nd:YAG laser in a power setting of 5–8 W (pulsed mode). This laser system is also very useful in patients with Morbus–Osler syndrome because of the common problem of bleeding from the oral cavity. Furthermore, there is a potential interest because of the aesthetic possibilities of these systems. The Er:YAG and the CO_2 laser should not be used for this kind of surgical treatment because the insufficient absorption and the penetration depth of the wavelengths of these lasers.

Drug-Induced Gingival Overgrowth

The surgical removal of gingival overgrowth using the CO_2 laser has been reported. There is no doubt that with this system the excision is comfortable and easy (very often using topical anesthesia). Cyclosporine-, nifedipine-, and hydantoin-induced gingival overgrowths can be excised relatively quickly with the CO_2 laser. Sometimes the high-pulsed CO_2 laser or a combination of scalpel excision and laser coagulation in a defocused mode for ablation is recommended. A periodontal pack and pain killers are not necessary after the laser treatment.

Tattoos and Pigmented Lesions

In patients with discoloration of the gingival tissues and a gummy smile, the removal of the gingival staining from the buccal gingival areas is sometimes indicated for aesthetic reasons. In such instances the CO_2 laser may be used successfully in an ablative mode. For the removal of pigmented lesions it is necessary to differentiate between hyperpigmentation and tumor before the use of laser. A biopsy is sometimes very useful to avoid postoperative complications, such as tumor irradiation. In dermatology, tattoos have been removed using dye lasers and Nd:YAG lasers, as they have been used in the oral cavity for removal of amalgam tattoos from the oral mucosa. In such applications the overheating of the tissues may result in postoperative pain as well as tissue damage and scar tissue formation.

Leukoplakia

The CO_2 laser has been used for the removal of leukoplakias for many years and different groups of clinicians have documented its long-term success. Specifically, a biopsy is necessary before the surgical excision. For wider lesions total excision of the leucoplakia is recommended with the CO_2 laser in a noncontact focused mode. As an alternative, the Er:YAG laser can be used for this clinical indication because the penetration depth of the CO_2 and the Er:YAG laser is not very high and light tissues without pigmentation better absorb the light in these wavelengths. Sometimes it is not possible to excise the white lesion totally and to examine it histopathologically because localization is very difficult to remove in toto. In such instances ablation and vaporization of the lesion is indicated. Close postoperative follow up of the patient is mandatory to document any recurrence or the possibility of cellular differentiation to a carcinoma in situ or a squamous carcinoma.

Small sized leukoplakias can also be removed using the defocused Nd:YAG or diode laser. It is of clinical relevance to avoid thermal damage when using these laser wavelengths to irradiate the oral tissues.

Peri-Implant Gingival Overgrowth

Excision of peri-implant gingival overgrowth is similar to the common gingivectomy in the periodontal tissues. The main problem of laser application in such regions is the absorption of the energy by the surface of the implant resulting in melting of the titanium and overheating. The CO_2, the diode (810 nm and 980 nm) as well as the Er:YAG laser may be used effectively to reduce the bacteria on the implant surface. This is of great importance in clinical cases with peri-implantitis, where the implant surface is decontaminated with the laser, and finally, the lost peri-implant tissues will be reconstructed by augmentation with graft materials. The Nd:YAG laser causes extensive melting and damage of the implant surface pattern and for this reason this kind of laser should be avoided in the field of implantology.

References

Horch HH, Gerlach KL, Schaefer HE. CO_2 laser surgery of oral premalignant lesions. *Int J Oral Maxillofac Surg* 1986;15:19–24.
Nakamura Y, Hossain M, Hirayama K, Matsumoto K. A clinical study on the gingival melanin pigmentation with the CO_2 laser. *Lasers Surg Med* 1999;25:140–147.

Pick RM, Pecaro BC, Silberman CJ. The laser gingivectomy. The use of the CO_2 laser for the removal of phenytoin hyperplasia. *J Periodontol* 1985;56:492–496.

Pick RM, Pecaro BC. Use of the CO_2 laser in soft tissue dental surgery. *Lasers Surg Med* 1987;7:207–213.

Poetke M, Philipp C, Berlien HP. Flashlamp-pumped pulsed dye laser for hemangiomas in infancy: Treatment of superficial vs. mixed hemangiomas. *Arch Dermatol* 2000; 136:628–632.

Romanos GE, Nentwig GH. Present and future of lasers in oral soft tissue surgery: clinical applications. *J Clin Laser Med Surg* 1996;14:179–184.

Roodenburg JL, Panders AK, Vermey A. Carbon dioxide laser surgery and oral leukoplakia. *Oral Surg Oral Med Oral Pathol* 1991;71:670–674.

White JM, Chaudhry SI, Kudler JJ, et al. Nd:YAG and CO_2 laser therapy of oral mucosal lesions. *J Clin Laser Med Surg* 1998;16:299–304.

Index

Entries are cross-referenced to their differential diagnoses. Numbers in *italics* refers to tables.